Mental Health Care for People of Diverse Backgrounds

Mental Health Care for People of Diverse Backgrounds

Edited by

Julia D Buckner

Assistant Director, Anxiety and Behavioral Health Clinic
Doctoral Candidate
FSU Psychology Clinic
Department of Psychology
Florida State University

Yezzennya Castro

Doctoral Candidate
FSU Psychology Clinic
Department of Psychology
Florida State University

Jill M Holm-Denoma

Doctoral Candidate
FSU Psychology Clinic
Department of Psychology
Florida State University

Thomas E Joiner, Jr

Director, FSU Psychology Clinic
The Bright-Burton Professor
Department of Psychology
Florida State University

Radcliffe Publishing
Oxford • Seattle

Radcliffe Publishing Ltd
18 Marcham Road
Abingdon
Oxon OX14 1AA
United Kingdom

www.radcliffe-oxford.com
Electronic catalogue and worldwide online ordering facility.

British Library Cataloguing in Publication Data

A catalogue record for this book is available from the British Library.

ISBN-10: 1 84619 094 0
ISBN-13: 978 1 84619 094 0

Typeset by Egan Reid Ltd, Auckland, New Zealand
Printed and bound by Biddles Ltd, King's Lynn, Norfolk, UK

Contents

To my family – Mom, Dad, Matt, Nathaniel, Lisa, and Lee – for their love and support (Julia).

My family, and my co-therapists who always work their hardest to deliver high quality services to people from all walks of life (Jill).

My family for their support, and my clients in Quincy for all they have taught me (Yezzennya).

To my two families – Zekey, Malachi, and Graciela, and FSU Psychology – though one is more important to me than the other, both are diverse and thriving (Thomas).

Acknowledgments

The efforts of the PhD students and the professors at Florida State University (FSU) Psychology have transformed the department's clinic into an award-winning enterprise dedicated to training psychological trainees on the delivery of empirically supported mental health services for diverse populations. In addition to ensuring high quality training of graduate student therapists, our vision has been to provide top-notch research-based mental health services for the greater Tallahassee community in order to ameliorate psychopathology quickly, with a strong focus on relapse prevention. As a result, the therapists at the FSU Psychology Clinic obtain unique training in the delivery of mental health services for a wide range of clients.

FSU therapists receive this training through the diligent supervision of several outstanding supervisors, including Donald Kerr, PhD, Norman B Schmidt, PhD, Ellen Berler, PhD, and Natalie Sachs-Ericsson, PhD. Their superb supervision and attention to the culturally competent delivery of mental health services have made this book possible.

We would also like to acknowledge the clients whom we have had the honor to serve at the FSU Psychology Clinic. We have learned so much from them and it is because of them that this work is meaningful.

About the Editors

Julia D Buckner, MS, **Yezzennya Castro, MS**, and **Jill M Holm-Denoma, MS** are doctoral candidates in clinical psychology at the Florida State University (FSU). Each has administered psychological services at the FSU Psychology Clinic (where case material for the book was developed), and each has a track record of research productivity. All have engaged in regular mental health service provision with clients from a variety of backgrounds.

Buckner's work focuses on the etiology, maintenance, prevention, and treatment of anxiety disorders, particularly the co-occurrence of anxiety and substance use disorders in children and adults from a diverse range of cultural backgrounds. She has submitted over 10 manuscripts for publication in peer-reviewed journals. Further, Buckner has served as the Assistant Director of FSU's Anxiety and Behavioral Health Clinic. There, she has supervised graduate student therapists and coordinated treatment outcome studies exploring the efficacy of treatments for particular anxiety disorders. Buckner has received several awards for her work including the Ruth L Kirschstein National Research Service Award.

Castro's interests include the appropriateness of assessment instruments for use with racial/ethnic minorities, culturally appropriate mental health services provision, and antisociality in women. She has submitted several works in these areas, and maintains a dedication to enhancing graduate students' understanding and appreciation of issues of diversity through her involvement in committees charged with increasing students' exposure to issues and research related to cultural diversity in clinical science. Her dedication to underserved populations is apparent in her clinical experiences, which have consisted of providing assessment, treatment, and prevention services to clients with limited income, migrant farm worker families, and incarcerated youth.

Holm-Denoma's research focuses on the classification of eating disorders, risk factors for eating disorder symptom development among individuals from diverse cultural groups, and the overlap between eating and mood disorders. She has published 10 articles in peer-reviewed journals, and has accrued clinical experience in outpatient clinics, inpatient state hospitals, and juvenile corrections facilities. Holm-Denoma has received multiple awards for her research, including the Joseph and Ruth Matarazzo Award from the American Psychological Foundation and the Florida State University Graduate Student Research and Creativity Award.

Thomas E Joiner, Jr, PhD is the Bright-Burton Professor and Director, University Psychology Clinic, in the Department of Psychology at the Florida

State University. Dr Joiner's work is on the psychology and neurobiology of suicidal behavior, depression, and eating disorders. Author of over 300 peer-reviewed publications, Joiner is editor of *Clinician's Research Digest*. He has received numerous research awards, including the Guggenheim Fellowship and the Award for Distinguished Scientific Early Career Contributions from the American Psychological Association. Dr Joiner is author or editor of 11 books, including *Why People Die by Suicide*, which was published in 2006 by Harvard University Press.

List of Contributors

Michael D Anestis, BA
Graduate Student
FSU Psychology Clinic
Department of Psychology
Florida State University
Tallahassee, FL

Jessica S Brown, MS
Assistant Director, FSU Psychology Clinic, 2004–2005
Doctoral Candidate
Department of Psychology
Florida State University
Tallahassee, FL

Carla Counts-Allan, MS
Doctoral Candidate
FSU Psychology Clinic
Department of Psychology
Florida State University
Tallahassee, FL

Kathryn H Gordon, MS
Assistant Director, FSU Psychology Clinic, 2005–2006
Doctoral Candidate
Department of Psychology
Florida State University
Tallahassee, FL

Daniel L Hollar, BS
McKnight Doctoral Fellow
FSU Psychology Clinic
Department of Psychology
Florida State University
Tallahassee, FL

Lora Rose Hunter, BA
Graduate Student
FSU Psychology Clinic
Department of Psychology
Tallahassee, FL

Lara J Jakobsons, MS
Gubernatorial Fellow
FSU Psychology Clinic
Department of Psychology
Florida State University
Tallahassee, FL

Karla K Repper, MS
Pre-Doctoral Intern
FSU Psychology Clinic
Department of Psychology
Florida State University
Tallahassee, FL

Robert C Schlauch, BA
Graduate Student
FSU Psychology Clinic
Department of Psychology
Florida State University
Tallahassee, FL

Norman B Schmidt, PhD
Professor of Psychology
Director of Clinical Training
Director, Anxiety and Behavioral Health Clinic
Department of Psychology
Florida State University
Tallahassee, FL

Kendra R Tannenbaum, MS
Doctoral Candidate
FSU Psychology Clinic
Department of Psychology
Florida State University
Tallahassee, FL

Matthew C Waesche, BS
Graduate Student
FSU Psychology Clinic
Department of Psychology
Florida State University
Tallahassee, FL

LaRicka Wingate, MS
Doctoral Candidate
FSU Psychology Clinic
Department of Psychology
Florida State University
Tallahassee, FL

Kimberly A Van Orden, MS
Assistant Director, FSU Psychology Clinic, 2006–2007
Doctoral Candidate
Department of Psychology
Florida State University
Tallahassee, FL

CHAPTER 1

Introduction to Empirically Informed Mental Health Services for Diverse Populations

Yezzennya Castro, Jill M Holm-Denoma, and Julia D Buckner

The number of individuals who identify as Hispanic/Latino is growing at a rate that is approximately four times that of the general United States population,[1] and these populations are expected to double by 2050.[2] Currently, individuals who identify as Hispanic/Latino and African American comprise 13% and 12% of the total United States population, respectively, which makes them the nation's two largest ethnic/racial minority groups.[3]

Ethnic and racial minority groups are not the only diverse groups that have experienced significant growth in recent years. Diversity, as defined by the American Psychological Association,[4] "recognizes the broad scope of dimensions of race, ethnicity, language, sexual orientation, gender, age, disability, class status, education, religious/spiritual orientation, and other cultural dimensions" (pp. 8–9). Statistics regarding the presence of diverse groups are now vital in understanding the cultural makeup of the United States. For instance, it is estimated that approximately 5% of individuals in the United States over the age of 18 identify themselves as gay or lesbian, and the size of this population has increased substantially in the past 10 years.[5] Recent estimates suggest that approximately 19% of Americans have a physical, sensory, or mental disability.[6] The family structure in the United States is different today than it was decades ago as well. For example, today 27% of children live in a single-parent home, 6% of children live in households with unmarried parents, and 5% of children live in a household with neither of their parents.[7] The religious topography of the United States is also changing, such that the percentage of nonreligious people and people who identify with non-Christian religions is increasing, whereas the percentage of those who identify themselves as Christian is decreasing.[8]

MENTAL ILLNESS IN DIVERSE GROUPS

Although it is notable that a substantial portion of the United States population identifies with at least one distinct cultural group, it cannot be overlooked that people fundamentally differ very little in many important ways. Relevant to this book is the fact that, regardless of their cultural identity, people as a rule do not differ significantly in their vulnerability to mental illness. For instance, epidemiological studies have estimated that the annual prevalence rate of mental disorders for adults and children in the United States is 21%, regardless of race or ethnicity.[9] Epidemiological data on adults indicates a 28–39% lifetime prevalence of mental disorders in communities across the United States.[10] The *Diagnostic and Statistical Manual of Mental Disorders*, fourth edition, text revision (DSM-IV-TR)[11] notes that the worldwide prevalence rates for most disorders, including schizophrenia, mood disorders, and anxiety disorders vary minimally across cultures.

Given that vulnerability to mental illness generally is fundamentally similar for all individuals, it is interesting when differences in occurrence or severity of mental illness are found between cultural groups. For instance, higher rates of mood, anxiety, and substance use disorders, and elevated rates of suicidal thoughts have been documented in adult gay and lesbian samples when compared with heterosexual men and women.[12] Also, higher rates of depression have been documented in American-born youth of Mexican descent compared with non-Hispanic and native Mexican youths.[13,14] Other notable findings include the Swedish national registry's report that children from single-parent homes have twice the rate of mental illness when compared with children from two-parent homes,[15] and that individuals with mental retardation are more likely to experience psychiatric disorders than the general population.[16]

This is not to say that being a member of a particular cultural group in and of itself accounts for these findings; rather, these findings point to the phenomenon of differential risk among given populations. That is, certain diverse groups may be exposed differentially to phenomena that can serve as risk factors for mental illness for all human beings. For example, research has provided evidence that individuals of racial/ethnic minority groups are likely to experience life stressors at increased rates when compared with majority groups.[17] One such life stressor is the experience of discrimination. Williams *et al.*[18] reviewed 23 studies that examined the association between discrimination and various aspects of mental health. All of the studies reviewed, which focused on variables ranging from general happiness to depression and anxiety to psychosis, found a positive association between discrimination and mental health problems. Discrimination does not only affect people of ethnic and racial minority groups. For instance, the experience of discrimination has been documented as a factor that may account for the increased risk of mental health problems in gay and lesbian populations as well.[12]

Low socioeconomic status (SES) is another life stressor and a risk factor for mental illness. Individuals with relatively lower income are more likely to experience mood and anxiety disorders compared with a reference group.[19] In addition, parental income is a significant predictor of adolescent depression,[20] and poverty is a contributing cause of mental illness in gay and bisexual Latino men.[21] One must consider findings such as these in light of facts such as that ethnic/racial minority groups and individuals with developmental disabilities are proportionately overrepresented in low SES conditions compared with majority populations.[9,22] As a consequence, some diverse groups that have relatively high rates of members living in low SES conditions may be at increased risk of mental illness.

In what is arguably the best example of a stressor that is unique to a diverse population, studies of gay, lesbian, and bisexual youth find that the unique experience of "coming out" can be very distressing. Pilkington and D'Augelli[23] surveyed almost 200 youth and found that 67% held significant fears related to coming out to friends and family, and many (22%) feared verbal or physical victimization in reaction to disclosing their sexuality. This is yet another example of how a life stressor associated with a particular cultural group, and not membership of this diverse group itself, constitutes an elevated risk toward mental illness.

THE NEED FOR CULTURALLY APPROPRIATE MENTAL HEALTH SERVICES PROVISION

Thus far, we have documented that a substantial amount of the United States population identifies with at least one diverse cultural group and that individuals (regardless of cultural group) are vulnerable to mental illness. Furthermore, certain cultural groups can experience mental illness at differential rates, because membership in that group may result in the greater, more severe, or more frequent experience of phenomena that increase the risk of mental illness (e.g., discrimination, low SES). In addition, some groups may experience unique life stressors that may serve as risk factors for mental illness (e.g., coming out). Clearly, these data imply that these culturally relevant factors deserve serious consideration in the delivery of mental health services (i.e., assessment, diagnosis, and treatment processes). As such, mental health professionals need to be aware of those risk factors to which individuals may be differentially exposed as a function of their experiences as a member of a diverse cultural group. In fact, the American Psychological Association[4] acknowledges that its ethical code implies the need for knowledge of different cultures and skill in treating people of diverse backgrounds if one is to provide the most appropriate and effective care.

Many more concerns have recently surfaced regarding mental health services provision to clients of diverse backgrounds. First, government officials have stressed that we must improve access to mental health treatment for diverse populations. Recently, members of ethnic and racial minority groups were reported to be less likely than Caucasian people to receive needed mental health services, and when they did receive them, they were of relatively poor quality.[9] A variety of explanations for these disparities have been suggested. One reason for this inequality in access to treatment involves health insurance. Compared with Caucasian people, a much higher percentage of Hispanic/Latino and African

American people are uninsured: uninsured rates are 18% for Caucasians, 25% for African Americans, and 37% for Hispanic/Latinos.[9] In addition, as the chapters on service provision to racial and ethnic minorities will discuss, issues of actual and perceived racism and discrimination of mental health service providers, distrust of the mental health system, language barriers, and a host of other factors may influence the quality of service received by members of diverse groups.[17]

A second concern that must be addressed is how to improve the quality of mental health treatment that is provided to members of diverse groups.[9] In addition to providing empirically supported or informed treatment, it has been recommended that mental health professionals should strive to consider a client's age, gender, sexual orientation, religious affiliation, race, ethnicity, and intellectual ability in a culturally sensitive and competent manner when providing mental health services.[17] Consideration of these cultural factors may involve a focus on how they can contribute to differential risk, as discussed earlier. The following chapters will also argue that it is important to consider how these factors may influence treatment and the therapeutic process. Treatment acceptance, adherence, and effectiveness may depend on the extent to which the therapist and the treatment take into consideration cultural beliefs and practices. It is optimal for clinicians to strive to incorporate these practices into the treatment process.

Last, it is essential for researchers to contribute to the knowledge base regarding how mental disorders affect diverse populations. Currently, the amount and quality of research conducted with nonminorities greatly outweighs that conducted with minorities.[9] In addition, of the research available on mental health and diverse populations, the vast majority is focused on uncovering differential risk, and as a result, we know very little about the mediators of these differences, similarities across various groups, or about unique protective factors for diverse populations.[24] Finally, there is currently a dearth of treatment outcome research that includes significant numbers of individuals of diverse backgrounds.[25] Hall[25] and Sue[26] make the noteworthy observation that no current empirically supported treatment has been established as effective according to the American Psychological Association Division 12 Task Force Guidelines for any diverse group.

WHAT DOES AND DOES NOT CONSTITUTE CULTURALLY SENSITIVE MENTAL HEALTH SERVICES PROVISION

Although there is currently a pressing need for more knowledge about how to provide proper services to diverse populations, views differ on the best way to accomplish this goal. Some might argue that cultural differences are so vast that each would need a treatment plan that was specially designed and validated for use with a given cultural group only. This conceptualization is known as the emic approach to explaining behavior, and it stresses the differences between groups of people. A problem with this approach is that it ignores the many basic and important similarities shared by human beings, and thus does not allow for researchers to empirically examine which treatment and assessment approaches might work similarly well in individuals from a variety of backgrounds. In addition, a more pressing matter is that the emic approach does not take into account the finding that the population of individuals of diverse backgrounds and identities is growing, and thus presenting in heightened rates at community mental health clinics now. As such, the development of emic treatments may be more time-consuming, costly, and impractical. Specifically, waiting for the development of these treatments would also fail to inform clinicians about how to best serve their clients now.[26]

However, to assume that the current tools and treatment approaches that were developed largely on majority groups should be adequate for diverse populations, or to assume that our social experiences are the same regardless of cultural background or identity, is also inadequate. The consequence of this practice (i.e., the etic approach) is to deny the diversity known to exist between and within groups. Specifically, taking this approach in research or practice would result in a bias toward attending to only the similarities between groups (while overlooking the sometimes important differences) and thus disallowing advancement of any knowledge about the influence of culture on behavior.[25]

A more balanced and realistic approach to culturally sensitive mental health care is one that is neither emic nor etic, as well as one that considers culture as neither a variable too overwhelming to be effectively addressed, nor an irrelevant variable to be ignored. Rather, culturally sensitive mental health services provision should consider culture to be a worthwhile variable for study in terms of its potential to explain a client's behavior, and its potential to give insight to aspects of treatment that may need to be modified to be more acceptable to and effective for the client. In addition, clinicians should strive to engage in their investigation of cultural variables in a nonjudgmental way.[4] This tenet comprises the general premise of *culturally competent mental health services provision*.

Although various attempts have been made at defining cultural competence, the most widely accepted definition was first proposed by Sue and colleagues.[27] They outline three components of cultural competence. *Knowledge* addresses the need to learn about and understand the worldviews of other cultures; *attitudes/beliefs* refers to the need for mental health professionals to be aware of their own beliefs and attitudes about other cultures; and *skills* addresses the need to use culturally appropriate intervention and communication skills. In addition to defining the three dimensions of cultural competence (knowledge, attitude/beliefs, and skills), Sue[26] identified three practical indicators of these competencies that may be suitable for research: (i) culture-specific expertise, (ii) dynamic sizing, and (iii) scientific mindedness.

Culture-specific Expertise

Culture-specific expertise involves having "specific knowledge about the cultural groups with which [you] work, understanding sociopolitical influences, and possessing specific skills needed in working with culturally different groups"[26] (p. 446). According to this model, knowledge of language, traditions, common worldviews, and experiences is necessary to make effective use of therapists' skills in dynamic sizing and scientific mindedness (which are described in the next two sections). More specifically, knowledge about a culturally diverse client's background is necessary to generate informed hypotheses about the role of culture in the treatment process. In addition, exhibiting knowledge of the client's culture helps with rapport and increases the therapist's credibility.

Dynamic Sizing

Sue[26] uses this term to refer to several aspects of a therapist's ability to appropriately apply knowledge of the client's background, and the ability of a therapist to be aware of how their own culture, beliefs, and/or misconceptions about the client's background affect the therapy process. For example, therapists must be aware of when it is and is not appropriate to apply their knowledge of the client's culture to their particular client's behavior. In addition, mental health care providers must be aware of how their own cultural background may affect their interpretation of client behavior. They must use their culture-specific knowledge to be aware of when the beliefs they hold about a client are factually true and when they are based on stereotypes.

Scientific Mindedness

Scientific mindedness refers to the use of the scientific method when investigating one's ideas of how the client's culture may affect assessment, diagnosis, and/or treatment. Sue[26] describes scientifically minded mental health care providers as those who use their culture-specific expertise to "form hypotheses rather than make premature conclusions about the status of culturally different clients, develop creative ways to test hypotheses, and act on the basis of acquired data" (p. 445). The main benefit of scientific mindedness is that it protects clinicians from acting on their personal judgments, which will be inevitably influenced by potentially erroneous beliefs or stereotypes about the client's culture.

Sue[26] emphasizes that these three factors are distinct and can exist independent of each other. For example, one can have a great deal of culture-specific expertise but lack skill in dynamic sizing or scientific mindedness. Use of one or two of the three factors in our interactions does not a culturally competent therapist make; rather awareness of all three facets of cultural competence, and repeated practice in use of all three is the best way to ensure that interactions with clients are culturally sensitive interactions. It is also important to understand that cultural competence is not a label that clinicians should award themselves at an arbitrary endpoint – they cannot take a class on culturally sensitive mental health care or read a book (although that is a start) and deem themselves culturally competent when the task is complete. Rather, it is a lens through which clinicians should attempt to view themselves, their clients, and their world. In addition to making a determined to effort to wear the lens, mental health care providers must expect to be constantly adjusting the lens with new knowledge, new skills, and new insights if they are to maintain it in focus.

ABOUT THE BOOK

This book has been created in an effort to meet several goals. First, it consolidates the extant theoretical and empirical literature on cultural issues that may affect the delivery of mental health care services across a variety of diverse populations. Thus it will serve as a comprehensive resource for mental health care providers to use when treating clients from diverse populations by allowing for easy access to information relevant to the provision of mental health services. Second, clinicians' use of this book as a guide for practicing culturally sensitive mental health care within an empirically informed framework will undoubtedly improve the quality of care that is given. Third, although this book addresses issues of culture relevant to the two largest ethnic/racial minorities in the United States (Hispanic/Latino and African American populations), it is unique in that it also addresses concerns relevant to topics that may have been previously overlooked in discussions of diversity. Specifically, this book addresses issues relevant to nontraditional families, individuals with developmental disabilities, and the role of an individual's religion or sexual orientation in therapy. Fourth, by consolidating information on these diverse populations into one resource, this book uniquely contributes to the current knowledge base regarding mental health provision to a wide range of individuals. Finally, it provides concrete examples of interactions with clients during the assessment, diagnosis, and treatment processes within a culturally competent and empirically informed framework.

The information contained in the following chapters is intended for individuals with many levels of clinical training and is therefore appropriate for trainees in psychology and psychiatry, as well as experienced mental health providers. The chapters contain information relevant to assessment, diagnosis, and treatment of individuals from diverse populations. Case studies have been included to illuminate and enliven the material. In this book, we strive to provide guidance regarding the practice of cultural sensitivity and competence in six diverse groups. The first three chapters will examine the cultural issues that may affect psychological services for African Americans, Hispanics/Latinos, and gay, lesbian, and bisexual individuals. The second half of the book will examine cultural sensitivity with regard to working with families, the role of religion in treatment, and working with individuals with a dual diagnosis of developmental disorders.

Each chapter begins by first identifying the salient cultural issues specific to the population of interest. We have already demonstrated above that there exists a notable amount of research on many basic cultural, social, and psychological factors that are relevant to diverse populations. It is likely that the mental health community has experienced ways in which empirical findings are discernible at the level of the individual client and are therefore relevant to practice. Indeed, the authors of these various chapters have noted clinical experience in which they have encountered the need to address culturally relevant issues. The authors draw from their own clinical experience to identify how specific cultural issues may manifest and potentially affect the assessment, diagnosis, and treatment of clients. The book intends to provide the reader with clear and realistic examples of how issues of culture or background may manifest through the use of case studies based on interactions with clients that the authors have actually experienced. By delineating examples from "real life" we hope to illuminate for the clinician those nuances of the treatment process that may have previously been overlooked as the result of hesitancy to acknowledge cultural differences.

Second, each chapter contains an extensive review of the existing literature to examine the theoretical and empirical evidence regarding the influence of culture on assessment, diagnosis, and treatment of each chapter's target population. This section includes both the identification of relevant cultural factors and the suggestions that have been previously offered to address these issues. This portion of each chapter is intended to serve as a reference concerning which cultural factors are known empirically to be relevant to the mental health of a given population so that the clinician can more efficiently create hypotheses about cultural influences on the behavior of the individual client. Third, a comprehensive case example is provided to illustrate how mental health providers may test their hypotheses regarding the client and to serve as a model for interacting with diverse clients in a culturally sensitive and appropriate manner. Finally, in order to encourage continued advancement of our knowledge of culture in therapy, each chapter offers suggestions for future research based on the authors' clinical experiences and the existing empirical evidence.

CHAPTER 2

The Assessment, Diagnosis, and Treatment of Psychiatric Disorders in Hispanic/Latino Clients

Lara J Jakobsons, and Julia D Buckner

According to population projections, Hispanic/Latino individuals will comprise 25% of the total United States population by 2050.[1] Given that the Hispanic/Latino population has become one of the fastest growing ethnic groups in the United States, clinicians are even more likely to treat people of Hispanic/Latino origin than they were in previous decades. Due in part to these changing demographics, it is crucial that mental health professionals are informed in the ways cultural issues can affect the assessment, diagnosis, and treatment of Hispanic/Latino clients. Although the overall rates of most psychiatric disorders in Hispanic/Latinos people are generally similar to those of non-Hispanic/Latino Caucasian populations,[2,3] the underlying causal mechanisms may differ between these groups. There are a number of factors that may place Hispanic/Latino individuals at increased risk for developing stress and subsequent mental health problems.[3,4] This chapter will outline cultural factors that may affect the assessment, diagnosis, and treatment of Hispanic/Latino clients.

Before discussing cultural competence when treating Hispanic/Latino clients, several remarks are in order regarding terminology. Specifically, the term "race" frequently refers to individuals of certain categories (e.g., Caucasian, black or African American) and individuals of Hispanic origin (e.g., Mexican, Cuban, Puerto Rican) are included in other race categories.[5] When referring to ethnicity, we are referring to either Hispanic or non-Hispanic individuals and this chapter is concerned with the Hispanic ethnic group. Although the United States Census Bureau states that Hispanics may be of any race, one caveat for this chapter is that we view the term "Hispanic" as usually referring to people of Spanish and Caribbean decent and the term "Latino" usually referring to people of Latin American descent. Thus, the two terms will be combined when used in this chapter in an effort to be as inclusive as possible. Also, due to the great within-group heterogeneity in Hispanic/Latinos cultures, another important caveat for the chapter is that differences may exist in the generalizability of research findings for the assessment, diagnosis, and treatment of specific Hispanic/Latino subgroups.

Psychological issues related to poverty are particularly salient for this population. To illustrate, in 2002, the Hispanic/Latino population represented 24% of the population living in poverty, and 21% of Hispanics/Latinos were living in poverty compared with 7% of the Caucasian population.[6] Hispanic/Latino workers also earned less than their Caucasian counterparts. Further, low socioeconomic status (SES) is associated with increased risk for depression among Hispanic/Latino college students.[7]

Limited education may serve as an additional barrier to treatment for Hispanic/ Latino individuals, as more than 2 in 5 Hispanics/Latinos aged 25 and older have not graduated from high school.[6] Concurrently, among Mexican American individuals, low educational achievement is correlated with depressive symptoms.[8]

Other factors that require further examination are a Hispanic/Latino person's risk for mental health problems as it relates to acculturative stress and the experience of discrimination. First, it is necessary to distinguish acculturative stress from acculturation, as confusion between the constructs has confounded findings about psychological distress in relation to acculturation.[9] Acculturative stress[10] specifically refers to stress resulting from the acculturative process, whereas acculturation is more broadly defined as the process of changes that individuals and groups experience when they come in contact with a new culture.[11] Importantly, there is a relation between levels of acculturative stress and mental health problems, such as depression.[9,12] Further, discrimination may be related to increased distress in Hispanic/Latino populations, as a positive correlation has been found between perceived discrimination and post-traumatic stress disorder (PTSD) symptoms in Hispanics/Latinos.[13] Other concerns with this population are language barriers and cultural differences in symptom patterns, exemplified by the presence of culture-bound syndromes in individuals of Hispanic/Latino origin.[14]

In addition, the Hispanic/Latino population underutilizes mental health services[15] and is less likely to take antidepressant medication in comparison with Caucasian clients.[16] There is also evidence that at least some Hispanic/Latino clients who do seek mental health services may limit self-disclosure during treatment.[17] Another obstacle is limited access to health care, as 37% of the Hispanic/ Latino population is uninsured.[18] Overall, these findings underscore the many barriers Hispanic/Latino clients may face related to treatment.

When treating Hispanic/Latino clients, the competence of clinicians can be increased through culture-specific expertise.[19] One way to achieve this is by possessing and utilizing knowledge of different concepts that commonly exist in the Hispanic/Latino culture. Cultural themes, such as *familismo, personalismo, respeto, marianismo, machismo, spiritualismo,* and *fatalismo* are important Hispanic/Latino values and practices. *Familismo* is described as the importance of prioritizing family and valuing close relationships among family members. *Personalismo* refers to valuing or building interpersonal relationships and using a warm, personal tone, and *respeto* reflects the expectation of others to show respect. Regarding gender roles, two cultural concepts may affect psychological services: *marianismo*, a woman's sense of selflessness and self-sacrifice; and *machismo*, a man's responsibility to protect and provide for the family. Hispanic/Latino culture also emphasizes a strong sense of spiritualism, *spiritualismo*, and a sense of destiny or that an event is "God's will", *fatalismo*. In addition to this culture-specific expertise, dynamic sizing (i.e., the therapist's ability to place the client's behavior in the proper cultural context) and scientific mindedness (i.e., the use of the scientific method when investigating one's ideas of how a client's culture may affect the therapeutic process) may translate into more efficacious psychological services.[19]

CLINICAL OBSERVATIONS
Assessment

Accurate assessment is the backbone of the delivery of appropriate psychological services. In our clinical experience, two important concerns arise when providing culturally competent assessment to Hispanic/Latino clients: language and the interpretation of equivalence for Hispanic/Latino clients on measures standardized on largely Caucasian populations. For example, an 18-year-old Mexican American woman, Elena, sought treatment for depression at our outpatient community clinic. The clinician was mindful that language can potentially affect the expression of symptoms and therefore asked Elena if she was proficient in Spanish and English. Since Elena endorsed proficiency in both languages, the clinician had to decide which language to use when conducting therapy. The clinician resolved this by simply asking Elena in which language she preferred to converse during treatment. As Elena stated she preferred English, the clinician administered the assessments and conducted treatment in English. By thoroughly assessing her client's language background and preference the clinician enhanced both the accuracy of her assessment and the strength of the therapeutic alliance.

Another cultural issue of importance in Elena's case was the interpretation of assessment instruments that are primarily standardized on Caucasian populations. One of the instruments that Elena completed in English was the Minnesota Multiphasic Personality Inventory-2 (MMPI-2).[20] Elena's profile indicated only a significantly elevated L scale. Following standard interpretation of the MMPI-2, the clinician might conclude that Elena's profile was similar to test-takers who display an overly virtuous self-presentation. However, this clinician was aware of research that has demonstrated a tendency for Hispanic/Latinos groups to obtain higher mean L scores in comparison with Caucasian groups.[21] Using scientific mindedness, the clinician formed two hypotheses from her profile: (i) Elena was attempting to make a socially desirable presentation or (ii) there was a cultural difference in her response style. By testing different hypotheses rather than forming an assumption about culturally diverse clients' performance, Elena's clinician was equipped to more accurately assess Elena's symptomatology.

Diagnosis

Clinicians must also allow cultural competence to guide diagnostic decisions. Differences in the experiences of Hispanic/Latino clients may or may not result in differential symptom presentations compared with non-Hispanic Caucasian clients. Therefore, a clinician can be most effective with culturally diverse clients if he or she is able to create an environment in which clients are comfortable discussing cultural issues, so that these issues can also be assessed for relevance to the presenting problem. Further, the clinician must be mindful of diagnostic criteria and ways in which a particular disorder may or may not be differentially expressed in Hispanic/Latino clients.

To illustrate, Jose, a Mexican immigrant, sought treatment at our clinic for anxiety symptoms. During the diagnostic assessment, Jose stated that he avoided contact with non-Hispanic Caucasian people due to the racism he has experienced in the United States. However, upon further probing, Jose's therapist was able to determine that Jose also avoided social situations in which he knew there would be no Caucasian people present, due to a fear of being embarrassed or ridiculed. Thus, his avoidance was the result of a fear of negative evaluation that is characteristic of a specific anxiety condition: social anxiety disorder (SAD). In other words, through careful probing by a therapist competent in dynamic sizing,[19] it was determined that by avoiding Caucasian people, as well as most other social interactions, Jose was avoiding social anxiety-provoking situations. His clinician was thus able to accurately diagnose Jose's condition and develop an effective treatment plan.

Treatment

In our clinical experience, we have noted at least two primary concerns regarding the treatment of Hispanic/Latino clients. First, given specific cultural differences between Hispanic/Latino and Caucasian groups, the treatments developed and evaluated for Caucasian populations may not be as effective for at least some Hispanic/Latino clients as they are for Caucasian clients. Second, some Hispanic/Latino clients may demonstrate a mistrust of mental health professionals that could hinder the therapeutic alliance, thereby impeding treatment. To address these issues, therapists in our clinic strive to provide a value-free environment so that individuals from all backgrounds can feel comfortable enough to adhere to treatment. We have found that the use of empirically informed treatments, combined with the application of the principles of self-determination theory (SDT)[22] (e.g., empathy, choice provision, rationale provision), results in the successful recruitment and retention of Hispanic/Latino clients.

Our success with this population suggests that many of the techniques that comprise empirically supported treatments are culturally sensitive. For example, Milagros, a 25-year-old woman originally from Puerto Rico, presented at our clinic for the treatment of SAD, public speaking type. Milagros' case was assigned to a non-Hispanic/Latina Caucasian woman and a traditional cognitive-behavioral therapy (CBT) protocol[23] was used. Initial sessions focused on teaching Milagros to identify negative automatic thoughts regarding her fear of negative evaluation. The remaining sessions focused primarily on exposure exercises aimed at providing disconfirming evidence to challenge her automatic thoughts and to encourage habituation of the physiological anxiety reactions that Milagros experienced during public speaking. The majority of the in-session exposure exercises conducted with Milagros involved repeated behavior speech tasks. Consistent with the principles of SDT, the therapist used choice provision, encouraging Milagros to choose the topics of her in-session exercises. Milagros often chose cultural issues as the topics of her speeches, including topics such as racial and cultural differences in women's rights in America and cultural differences between Christmas traditions in the United States versus those practiced in Puerto Rico. After 12 sessions, Milagros' SAD remitted and she and her clinician mutually agreed on termination.

This case example addressed both treatment concerns outlined above. Milagros' successful completion of a traditional CBT protocol resulting in remittance of her disorder suggests that CBT for SAD may require no modification for Hispanic/Latina clients. Her therapist's use of the principles of SDT created an environment in which Milagros was comfortable discussing cultural differences. This environment may have assuaged any mistrust Milagros had regarding treatment and strengthened the therapeutic alliance, increasing the likelihood that treatment would be efficacious. It is also noteworthy, however, that Milagros serves as just one example of the successful implementation of extant empirically supported treatments for use with Hispanic/Latino individuals; much more work is necessary to determine whether all empirically informed treatments are effective with this population.

Given the emphasis on interpersonal relationships in Hispanic/Latino cultures, it follows that treatments specifically focusing on interpersonal functioning may also be particularly effective. For example, Interpersonal Psychotherapy (IPT)[24] and Cognitive Behavioral Analysis System of Psychotherapy (CBASP)[25] emphasize interpersonal relationships. Similar to CBT, the client chooses situations on which to focus for both IPT and CBASP. Further, the client's values dictate the direction of these treatments (vs. the therapist's agenda which could be influenced by therapist culture, stereotypes, discrimination, etc.). CBASP in particular serves as a model of treatment in which the client's values drive treatment. The client is required in CBASP to present in each session with a completed homework assignment detailing an interpersonal interaction. The client first provides a brief description of this situation. Next, the client outlines the thoughts and behaviors in which he or she engaged during the interaction. Third, the client lists what they desired to achieve in the interpersonal interaction (i.e., the "desired outcome"). This desired outcome is generated by the client (not the therapist) and therefore reflects the choices of the client within their own cultural framework. Fourth, the client describes what actually happened. Lastly, the client is asked if they achieved the desired outcome and, if they did not, the client works with the therapist to remediate the thoughts and behaviors in which the client engaged.

Specifically, thoughts and behaviors are identified that can be implemented in future interpersonal interactions to increase the likelihood the client will obtain his or her desired outcome. Again, the remediated thoughts and behaviors originate from the client and therefore are more likely to be consistent with their cultural context; the thoughts are remediated in light of how to best achieve the desired outcome, which too, is generated within the client's own cultural framework.

THE CURRENT STATE OF THE LITERATURE
Assessment

As discussed above, there are several factors that may affect the assessment of Hispanic/Latino clients. Unfortunately, there is little research investigating which factors affect assessment of this population. However, as with any initial assessment, it is necessary to collect patient data on presenting problem, expectations for therapy, suicidality, work history, family composition and relationships, religious and spiritual beliefs, education, work history, SES, and functioning level. Careful assessment of family composition and relationships may be necessary with some clients, as interpersonal relationships are emphasized in Hispanic/Latino culture. In addition, the client's spiritual or religious values may also be relevant in the context of treatment, as a recent poll indicated that over 70% of the Hispanic/Latino population in the United States self-identified with the Catholic religion.[26] Given that Hispanics/Latinos are over represented in low SES and educational achievement groups (as discussed previously), related stressors that may impact a client's mental health and treatment (e.g., malnutrition, housing problems, poor medical care) should be thoroughly assessed.[27]

The limited existing literature suggests that more specific cultural factors, such as acculturation, acculturative stress, cultural conflicts, immigration history, minority status, and experiences with discrimination need to be assessed in Hispanic/Latino clients.[27–30] For example, the process of acculturation affects language, values, beliefs, and customs, and has been shown to be a significant factor in assessment of Hispanic/Latino clients.[31] It has been suggested that the process of acculturation leads to a weakening of cultural values of family, and thus diminishes protective factors related to resources and support.[32] Further, there is a relation between levels of acculturative stress and mental health problems.[9,12] Given these data, clinicians may choose to evaluate the role of acculturation in presenting symptomatology. Several measures that assess acculturation demonstrate adequate psychometrics, including the Multidimensional Acculturative Stress Inventory,[33] a measure of acculturative stress in adults of Mexican origin, and the Hispanic Stress Inventory,[34] a measure of psychosocial stress. The clinician can also ask the client's place of birth, and if applicable, the reason for immigration and number of years living in the United States

Language may affect the expression of pathology in Hispanic/Latino clients, complicating assessment. Inaccurate assessment can arise if a mental health care provider misinterprets the client's symptom expression.[35] It is therefore helpful to demonstrate scientific mindedness by assessing language background, proficiency, and preference.[29] For example, conducting treatment in English with a bilingual client may result in misinterpretation of the client's behaviors[36] or may limit the ability of the client to accurately express emotion,[37] which could result in inaccurate diagnostics. Moreover, the bilingual client may focus more on pronouncing English words accurately, rather than conveying meaningful content.[38] In contrast, if the clinician is not proficient in Spanish, an interpreter may be necessary or the client may be referred for services with a Spanish-speaking clinician. However, interpreters may create other challenges, such as the extra time spent translating, confidentiality issues, and errors made by untrained interpreters.[39] Unfortunately, given the limited research in this area, it is not yet possible to establish clear recommendations for bilingual clients regarding language usage. Nevertheless, one way to assess the appropriateness of a measure for a client is to simply ask the client if any items on a measure were unclear or difficult for them to understand, due to language or culture.

Another important concern regarding assessment in this population relates to the need for standardized measures in Spanish. It is important to determine whether measures developed in English contain the same meaning when translated into Spanish. Specifically, the clinician is recommended to use instruments in which translation (linguistic), conceptual (meaning), and metric equivalence from English to the Spanish language have been established. Translation equivalence may be demonstrated by translation (from English to Spanish), back translation (from Spanish to English), followed by comparison and revision.[40] Unfortunately, few measures meet these criteria, and few studies have examined whether measures developed in English and standardized on Caucasian populations contain the same meaning, linguistics, and metric calibration in Spanish.

There is preliminary empirical support for several Spanish and Portuguese-version assessment instruments. Clinical interviews that are available in Spanish include the Structured Clinical Interview for DSM-IV Axis I Disorders (SCID),[41] the Structured Clinical Interview for DSM-IV Personality Disorders (SCID-II),[42] the Diagnostic Interview Schedule (DIS)[43] and the Psychiatric Research Interview for Substance and Mental Disorders (PRISM).[44] Regarding symptom inventories, both the Beck Anxiety Inventory (BAI)[45] and Beck Depression Inventory (BDI)[46] have versions translated in Spanish[47,48] and the Eating Disorder Inventory (EDI)[49] has been translated in Portuguese.[50] In general, there is some empirical support for these measures. For instance, adequate psychometrics on the Portuguese version of the EDI have been obtained.[50]

However, there are limitations to these measures. For example, although the Spanish-version BDI has demonstrated good psychometric properties overall, one study indicated four items may not be accurately assessing depressive symptomatology among Hispanic/Latino clients.[51] Specifically, Spanish-speaking clients in this study were more likely to endorse items reflecting punishment, appearance, and tearfulness, and less likely to endorse ability to work. This potential bias may be due to the behaviors or beliefs being specific to a culture rather than depressive symptoms, or this propensity may simply be an artifact of translation.[51] Regarding the item, "I feel like I am being punished," for instance, it is possible that endorsement by Spanish-speaking clients may reflect a cultural-specific notion of *fatalismo* or pessimism. In addition, there may be possible language and acculturation differences in response style on the Spanish version of the MMPI-2.[52-54] Thus, further research is warranted to ensure semantic equivalence for Spanish-speaking populations.

It is also necessary to determine whether current assessment measures demonstrate adequate psychometric properties and utility for English-speaking Hispanic/Latino clients. For example, initial data suggest that the use of the BDI and BAI yields psychometric properties comparable with those exhibited in Caucasian samples.[55] A meta-analysis of MMPI/MMPI-2 studies revealed minor differences between Caucasian and Hispanic/Latino groups and the Hispanic/Latino group was not portrayed "unfairly" as more pathological.[21] However, aggregate effect sizes indicated higher scores on the L (Lie) scale and lower scores on scale 5 (Masculinity-Femininity) for Hispanic Latino men (mostly Mexican American) relative to the Caucasian group. A possible interpretation for the elevations on the L scale includes that Hispanic/Latino individuals may be attempting to make a socially desirable presentation. In contrast, a cultural difference in the response style of the Hispanics/Latino group may exist, possibly related to their strong cultural value of spiritualism,[56] or reluctance to admit personal distress, in comparison with African American and Caucasian counterparts.[13] The lower scale 5 scores, indicating heightened traditional masculine gender identification among Hispanic/Latino men, may be explained as denoting a cultural difference in response style (related perhaps to *machismo*) instead of psychopathology.[56] These data suggest there may be utility of current instruments for English-speaking Hispanic/Latino individuals but that modification in scale and/or interpretation may be necessary for some instruments.

Diagnosis

There is also a dearth of research examining whether the expression of psychopathology is affected by cultural influences. Although overall rates of psychiatric disorders in the Hispanic/Latino population appear to be similar to rates in Caucasian populations, some differential expression for specific disorders may exist. For example, depression appears to occur at a slightly higher rate in Hispanic/Latino adults and adolescents relative to Caucasian individuals.[3,14,57] Hispanic/Latino Americans also appear to have higher rates of PTSD than Caucasian and African American individuals.[13] Further, among individuals with PTSD, it appears that Hispanic/Latino clients present with elevated rates of dissociative symptoms relative to other groups.[58] One interpretation regarding the increased rates of PTSD is that Hispanic/Latino individuals respond to distress with avoidance (a hallmark feature of anxiety disorders) more so than other cultures.[13] Avoidance may be the result of high religiosity; for instance, *fatalismo* and religious beliefs in the Hispanic/Latino culture are associated with increased PTSD avoidance symptoms.[59] In addition, lower social support, increased perceived racism, increased wishful thinking and self-blame coping, and increased peritraumatic dissociation (reactions that occur during or directly after the traumatic event) also appear related to elevated PTSD symptoms in the Hispanic/Latino population.[13] However, the nature of the relations between these factors and PTSD is unclear. For example, it is unclear if perceived racism is a cause or consequence of PTSD symptoms, and requires longitudinal research.[13]

When diagnosing Hispanic/Latino clients, it is also important to be mindful of the degree to which symptomatology varies within the broad Hispanic/Latino culture.[29] For instance, preliminary research suggests that Puerto Ricans living in New York have high rates of depression.[60] In contrast, Cuban Americans overall tend to have fairly low rates of depression.[61]

There also appears to be a relation between acculturative stress and symptomatology in the Hispanic/Latino population. Specifically, higher rates of depression, phobias, and substance use disorders (SUDs) have been found in Mexican Americans born in United States (who are assumed to be more acculturated) in comparison with those born in Mexico.[62-64] It may be that Mexican Americans born in the United States have higher expectations regarding education and income, and may be more likely to feel depressed when they do not reach their goals.[32,64] Further, heightened levels of acculturative stress predict depression and suicidal ideation in Mexican immigrants and second-generation Hispanic/Latino adolescents.[9,12] For example, one study found that Mexican American adolescent girls exhibited more depressive symptoms and negative cognitive styles, which were characterized by pessimism instead of fatalism, compared with non-Mexican American girls.[65] These results suggest that depressive symptoms in Mexican American adolescents may be produced by culturally specific pessimism that interacts with acculturative stress. Alternatively, positive expectations for the future, and elevated religiosity and perceived quality of social support, may buffer against levels of distress.[9,12]

Diagnosis of Hispanic/Latino clients is also complicated by the existence of culture-bound syndromes. A culture-bound syndrome is defined as a repetitive pattern of problematic experience and abnormal behavior often regarded as an "illness," which is usually delineated to certain local cultural areas or societies.[66] This syndrome may or may not relate to a specific DSM-IV diagnostic category. For example, *ataque de nervios* (attack of nerves) is a culture-bound syndrome characterized by trembling, uncontrollable shouting, attacks of crying, dissociative experiences, screaming uncontrollably, and fear.[66] This syndrome is manifested frequently among Latinos from the Caribbean (particularly Puerto Rican women) and individuals from Latin America. It should be noted that *ataques* is listed in the DSM-IV appendix on culture-bound syndromes. Although research on *ataques* in non-Hispanic/Latino populations is lacking, this syndrome suggests culturally relevant gaps in our current diagnostic criteria given that the current system does not capture these cultural differences in symptoms.[14]

Treatment

Unfortunately, few studies have investigated the effectiveness of empirically validated treatments for specific disorders for Hispanic/Latino clients. The good news is that the few studies that have been conducted suggest that at least some empirically validated treatments are effective for this population.

There is good evidence that CBT and IPT are promising treatments for depressive symptomatology in at least some Hispanic/Latino clients. For example, among 26 Puerto Rican women, five sessions of cognitive group therapy and of behavioral group therapy yielded decreased depressive symptomatology relative to a wait-list control condition.[67] The observed improvements persisted at a five-week follow-up assessment. In addition, in a comparison of the effectiveness of psychopharmacology, CBT, and community mental health care in a sample that was approximately 50% Hispanic/Latina, the data suggest that both CBT and medications are superior to community mental health.[68] Primary care interventions that utilize CBT have also been found to result in decreased depressive symptomatology relative to no-treatment and psychotropic medication management among African American and Hispanic/Latino clients at six months.[69] Further, Hispanic/Latino and African American clients maintain treatment gains at five-year follow-up that are comparable to treatment gains achieved by Caucasian clients.[70] A recent study found that IPT may also be effective in the treatment of depression among Hispanic/Latina adolescent girls in school clinic settings.[71] Relative to treatment as usual, the girls in the IPT condition demonstrated fewer clinician-reported depression symptoms, greater clinical improvement, greater decrease in clinical severity, better global functioning, and improved social functioning.

There is also evidence indicating that some existing interventions may be effective in preventing depression in at least some Hispanic/Latino populations. For instance, in a randomized controlled trial of a depression prevention course using CBT techniques in a sample that was approximately 25% Hispanic/Latino, individuals in the CBT condition had significantly reduced depressive symptomatology relative to the no-treatment condition at six-month follow-up.[72] Taken together, these data suggest that CBT may be an effective treatment and prevention for Hispanic/Latino clients with depressive symptomatology.

Fewer studies have been published investigating the effectiveness of treatments for anxiety disorders among Hispanic/Latino clients. To our knowledge, only one study has specifically examined the treatment of anxiety disorders in Hispanic/Latino clients.[73] In this investigation, CBT was utilized for the treatment of childhood anxiety and the findings indicate that Hispanic/Latino children fare as well as Caucasian children when CBT is used to treat anxiety. In a study in which the sample consisted of 41% Hispanics/Latino clients, group CBT was administered to children and adolescents.[74] Separate group sessions were conducted with the parents of these children and adolescents. Youths in the group CBT condition demonstrated significantly lower rates of anxiety diagnoses post-treatment and improvements were maintained at one-year follow-up assessments. Overall, the results of these two studies suggest that traditional CBT protocols can be as effective for Hispanic/Latino clients as for Caucasian clients in the treatment of anxiety conditions.

Some attention has been paid to the treatment of disruptive behaviors among Hispanic/Latino adolescents. Given the importance of folklore in some Hispanic/Latino cultures, one group of researchers has been working to develop and evaluate interventions utilizing folklore and story-telling in the treatment of behavioral problems among Puerto Rican American school children. One study was conducted on eighth and ninth graders and consisted of small group sessions in which the youths read biographies of heroic Puerto Rican adults.[75] This approach was chosen to both increase cultural sensitivity of the treatment of Puerto Rican youths and provide positive adult role models to this population. Compared with a control group consisting of eight sessions that met to discuss current events, the treatment condition demonstrated increased Puerto Rican identity and decreased trait anxiety (among eighth graders only). However, several limitations to this study make its findings difficult to interpret. For example, the treatment condition consisted of nearly twice as many sessions as the control group. In addition, the effect of the treatment on disruptive behaviors was not reported. Although promising, additional research is necessary before conclusions regarding the effectiveness of folklore treatment for Puerto Rican American adolescents with behavioral problems can be determined. A similar study was conducted on a younger age group (kindergarten to third grade) for the treatment of behavioral problems.[76] This study compared the Puerto Rican story-telling to an adapted (Puerto Rican/United States) folklore, an art/play condition, and no treatment. Clients in the Puerto Rican and adapted folklore conditions reported significantly fewer anxiety symptoms than the other two conditions. However, there were no long-term differences between conditions on measures of social adjustment or on behavior outcomes (e.g., disruptive behavior), indicating the utility of folklore treatments for disruptive behaviors in Puerto Rican children is questionable.

In examining the existing treatment outcome literature on the treatment of Hispanic/Latino clients, there are several noteworthy limitations deserving discussion. First, there may be differences between various Hispanic/Latino cultures that may affect treatment response, yet to our knowledge no studies have examined differential treatment response among different Hispanic/Latino groups. A second limitation is that most studies conduct treatment in English. However, Pina et al.[73] have found that individuals who speak English as a second language responded as well as native English speakers, suggesting that the observed treatment gains using English protocols could also be viewed as a strength and speak to the universality of treatments such as CBT. Third, although some treatment studies consisted of large numbers of Hispanic/Latino clients, many of them did not evaluate differences in treatment between the Hispanics/Latino and Caucasian groups[68] to determine if differential treatment outcomes occur, and if so, what variables moderate these differences. Fourth, only two studies have investigated treatments for anxiety disorders in Hispanic/Latino clients.[73,74] Although the findings of these preliminary studies are encouraging in that both individual CBT and group CBT were found to be effective treatments for this population, these studies were conducted on samples in which all anxiety disorders were collapsed across conditions. In other words, specificity of treatment for particular anxiety disorders has not been investigated among Hispanic/Latino clients. In addition, the extant research on anxiety treatments has been conducted on child and adolescent samples and future research is necessary to determine if CBT is an effective treatment for anxiety disorders among Hispanic/Latino adults.

Another important area of research relevant to the treatment of Hispanic/Latino clients examines ethnic matching between clinician and patient. One study suggests that Mexican Americans with lower levels of acculturation may prefer ethnically similar therapists and having a non-matched therapist may inhibit trust and self-disclosure.[17] However, Maramba and Hall's meta-analysis[77] indicated that ethnic match alone is a weak predictor of retention in therapy. In fact, results from one study indicate that Mexican Americans (regardless of level of acculturation) rated perceptions of cultural sensitivity in the clinician as one of the most significant variables, independent of patient's acculturation or clinician's ethnicity.[78] Overall, this research suggests that clinicians of all ethnicities can provide culturally competent treatment.

COMPREHENSIVE CASE ILLUSTRATION

To demonstrate the unique cultural issues with which Hispanic/Latino clients may present during assessment, diagnosis, and treatment, a case presentation follows. Gloria, a 53-year-old divorced Hispanic/Latina woman, who was bilingual in Spanish and English, was treated by a female, non-Hispanic/Latina Caucasian clinician. As discussed above, assessment consisted of the standard assessment used for all clients (presenting problem, suicidality, education, work history, family composition and relationships, religious and spiritual beliefs, etc.). In addition, the clinician was mindful of culture-related issues, such as immigration history, acculturation, and cultural role conflicts, as elaborated below.[28]

Gloria's presenting problem consisted of depressive symptoms and she hoped to learn coping skills for dealing with stress. Although current suicidal ideation was denied at intake, she endorsed past suicidal ideation, as well as having plans and preparations for suicide several weeks before. Thus, her suicide risk fell in the moderate range.[79] Following the suicide assessment, the clinician assessed Gloria's acculturation and language skills. She was born in Mexico and immigrated to the United States when she was 15 years old. Gloria was proficient in English and stated she preferred the assessment and treatment to be conducted in English. Gloria maintained a very close relationship with her parents in Mexico, her daughter, grandchildren, and four siblings (i.e., demonstrating *familismo*). In addition, she reported a few American friends and endorsed participation in American traditions (i.e., indicating fair acculturation). Gloria also reported that she had not completed college and indicated a limited work history (i.e., currently unemployed, as her ex-husband had previously provided for her). Gloria was a devout Catholic, attending church weekly and believing strongly that events reflected God's will (i.e., *fatalismo*).

Regarding Gloria's family and social history, at 22 years of age she married a non-Hispanic/Latino Caucasian man whom she described as very controlling and who drank alcohol frequently. They had a son and a daughter together. After 20 years of marriage, she divorced her husband due to his frequent infidelity. Her 19-year-old son, Miguel, had a 2-year-old son, John, and a 4-year-old daughter, Sara, both of whom lived with and were primarily cared for by Gloria.

The clinician used her culture-specific knowledge to inform assessment. Due to Gloria's proficiency in English, her functioning and symptoms were assessed using standard instruments in English. Gloria scored in the moderate range on the BDI, BAI, and Beck Scale for Suicide Ideation.[80] On the EDI, Gloria's scores fell in the clinical range on the Body Dissatisfaction and Perfectionism subscales. To assess if items on the measures were problematic, the clinician asked Gloria if any items were unclear or difficult to understand. This discussion helped the clinician decide that the measures appeared appropriate for her client as Gloria did not endorse confusion on any of the items and no inconsistencies in response pattern were observed.

To determine Gloria's diagnoses, the clinician administered the Mini International Neuropsychiatric Interview (MINI).[81] Since childhood, Gloria reported symptoms of depression and an inability to recall a time when she was happy. She complained of fluctuations in appetite, difficulty sleeping, lethargy, excessive guilt, difficulty making decisions, hopelessness, and suicidal ideation. Regarding her eating, Gloria reported frequent binge episodes in which she felt "out of control," several times per week. The binge episodes began during her divorce and were followed by a gain in weight. Since the time of her divorce, she began feeling that her body weight influenced how she viewed herself. Gloria met the DSM-IV criteria for major depressive disorder, dysthymic disorder, and eating disorder not otherwise specified.

In addition, Gloria reported several stressors, such as her unstable relationship with her son, who had a history of drug use, alcohol use, and violence. Further, she felt a great deal of bitterness toward her ex-husband and her interactions with him were usually unpleasant. Moreover, her granddaughter, Sara, was frequently displaying defiant behavior, which was an additional source of frustration.

In giving standard diagnostic feedback, the clinician provided Gloria with rationale for treatment and choice provision (i.e., SDT principles) following our clinic's protocol. Given that treatment of depression was prioritized, the clinician briefly described the empirically informed treatments available (CBT, IPT, and CBASP). The clinician and Gloria mutually agreed that CBASP, an empirically supported treatment for chronic depression, would be the best treatment for her at this time. Gloria expressed reservation about treating her binge episodes, so it was decided that they would be targeted once her depression was under control, if the binges were still present. Overall, although there is no controlled research on CBASP treatment with Hispanic/Latino populations, realistic expectations and mutual goals for therapy were set within an empirically informed framework, with which Gloria stated she was comfortable. It was decided that progress in treatment would be assessed through the routine administration of the BDI, BAI, EDI, and Beck Suicide Scale (BSS).

Throughout treatment, the clinician encouraged Gloria's language style and usage of *dichos* while learning problem solving strategies in CBASP. *Dichos* are proverbs, folk sayings, or metaphors in the Spanish language that are often utilized by individuals from Hispanic/Latino cultures. Preliminary research suggests such benefits of *dichos* include helping the client reframe problems and increasing the client's motivation for treatment.[82,83] Gloria's use of *dichos* achieved effects similar to those observed in the literature. For instance, Gloria frequently dwelled on her ex-husband's infidelity and his younger girlfriends. During one session, Gloria was applying the CBASP framework and one of her helpful thoughts was the *dicho*, "Lo que pasó voló," which translates to "There's no use in crying over spilled milk" or "Let bygones be bygones."[84] This proverb especially helped her to "move on" and focus on the present, instead of the past and her ex-husband. Gloria reported that the usage of *dichos* helped her "to open up" and feel more comfortable sharing experiences with the clinician.

Relatedly, another characteristic of Hispanic/Latino culture, *personalismo* (i.e., relating in a warm, personal tone) was used by both Gloria and her clinician. For example, Gloria enjoyed bringing in pictures of her family to show the clinician. The clinician found that these more personal interactions increased rapport and Gloria's motivation for treatment.

Similar to other clients who are of low SES, Gloria had limited resources. Outside her family, Gloria had a small social network and her clinician encouraged her to join a community-based group. Through the group, Gloria met a number of friends who were supportive of her treatment, and increased her social interactions. Relatedly, Gloria could not afford a baby-sitter during the therapy sessions and therefore had to arrange for her daughter to watch the grandchildren. Treatment progress with Gloria was slightly slower than with other clients because she occasionally could not attend weekly therapy sessions if her daughter was unavailable for baby-sitting. More specifically, the clinician showed understanding during treatment when Gloria canceled an appointment with at least 24-hour notice, due to her daughter's unavailability. Thus, the clinician demonstrated cultural competence by being aware of the obstacles that individuals with limited financial resources face.

In general, the therapist was able to incorporate such cultural values as *respeto* into the CBASP framework. This treatment appeared to create a non-judgmental environment in which Gloria was able to discuss cultural issues, thus reflecting the clinician's cultural competence. For example, within the CBASP framework, Gloria was able to maintain her *fatalismo* while realizing that only she could have control over her thoughts, behaviors, and desired outcomes. This realization positively influenced the outcomes of a situation. As a result, CBASP helped her discover that she always had choices in situations.

In addition, the CBASP framework accommodated Gloria's *familismo* through its emphasis on interpersonal relationships. Cultural issues, such as *marianismo*, *machismo*, and *respeto* with her son, ex-husband, and granddaughter were targeted using CBASP. Gloria valued the cultural concept of being the caregiver when she was married and relinquished the task of providing financially to her husband. As a result, her lifelong goal was to be a home-maker. During therapy, Gloria realized that she was a divorced woman who was solely caring for her two grandchildren, which necessitated her taking on the role of financial provider and coming to terms with her new nontraditional role. Moreover, Gloria held the belief that she should be self-sacrificing in her relationships with her ex-husband, son, and grandchildren. Likewise, she experienced much frustration when she performed selfless behaviors for her family without any appreciation or recognition. CBASP enabled her to achieve realistic and attainable desired outcomes and expectations in these interpersonal situations. Gloria was also better able to set boundaries in relationships and realize it was her choice to perform selfless acts for her family, and that she could not control others' responses, which decreased her frustration. In sum, CBASP aided Gloria in coming to terms with cultural conflicts regarding gender role expectations.

These therapeutic gains were further confirmed by Gloria's scores on assessment measures, which were periodically administered to monitor treatment progress. In particular, during the sixth therapy session, a significant reduction in Gloria's symptoms was evident, as her BAI, BDI, and BSS scores all fell to within the mild or normal range. This decrease in her symptoms was maintained for 12 weeks, during which time her scores consistently remained in the normal range. In addition, Gloria's scores on the EDI subscales fell to within the normal range during the ninth session and were maintained during the remainder of treatment. Gloria attended a total of 12 therapy sessions over 26 weeks, and at termination the BDI, BAI, and BSS were readministered. Her scores were in the normal range across all measures, and Gloria denied suicidal ideation, plans, or preparations. Furthermore, conflicts between Gloria and her son, granddaughter, and ex-husband were resolved. Consequently, the new skills learned from CBASP generalized to her binge eating, as she felt more in control of her emotions and eating. Specifically, Gloria lost 5.8 kg (13 lb) and had not binged since her sixth therapy session. She also began eating small meals throughout the day and exercising several times a week. Gloria reported that her self-esteem increased, expectations for her ideal weight decreased, and she felt happy with her body. In addition, she began wearing make-up and took more of an interest in her clothes. For the first time in many years, she felt that she was "ready" to meet a new partner. Lastly, Gloria began a day-care center in her home and successfully came to terms with her gender role conflict by acknowledging that her "mother" role required her to be a financial provider to her grandchildren.

CONCLUSIONS AND FUTURE DIRECTIONS

The clinical and empirical data presented in this chapter point to exciting avenues of future work in the assessment, diagnosis, and treatment of Hispanic/Latino clients. Specifically, the chapter advocated assessing standard areas during intake, in addition to considering culture-specific issues such as acculturation, acculturative stress, immigration history, and language proficiency. Although a few studies have examined the psychometric properties and utility of assessment instruments with Hispanic/Latino clients (e.g., MMPI-2, BDI, BAI), further examination of additional measures and clinical interviews is necessary. Moreover, future research is needed to study the translation and interpretation equivalence of the Spanish versions of instruments, as well as the standardization and validation of the use of such instruments in Hispanic/Latino populations.

Related to diagnostics, research indicates that despite similar rates of psychopathology generally, the Hispanic/Latino population may be more vulnerable to mood and anxiety disorders relative to Caucasian populations. Future work is necessary to identify risk factors for this differential symptom expression as well as to investigate diagnostic prevalence rates within the different Hispanic/Latino subgroups.

Regarding treatment, emerging evidence suggests that CBT is an effective treatment for anxiety and depressive conditions among Hispanic/Latino clients. However, given the dearth of treatment outcome data, much more research is necessary to evaluate the effectiveness of CBT for other disorders. In addition, as the majority of the research that has been conducted has focused on anxiety in youth and depression in adults, further research is necessary to ascertain whether the positive treatment outcomes observed for these disorders also occurs in other disorders and across all ages. Also, although it is necessary to determine whether or not treatments work for Hispanic/Latino clients, an equally important question is how treatments work for these clients.[85] To this end, additional research is necessary to identify factors that moderate and mediate treatment change (e.g., such as cultural matching between client and therapist, discrimination, SES, education, acculturation, English proficiency).

Furthermore, there is still good reason to evaluate treatments tailored to the cultural concerns of Hispanic/Latino clients. Given the emphasis on interpersonal relationships in Hispanic/Latino cultures, it follows that treatments that specifically focus on interpersonal functioning may be particularly effective. For example, both IPT and CBASP emphasize interpersonal functioning. Although there is some evidence that IPT may be effective in the treatment of depression in Hispanic/Latina patients,[71] much more research is necessary before IPT can be recommended as a treatment of choice for Hispanic/Latino groups for depression and/or other diagnoses. Unfortunately, we know of no studies that have investigated the effectiveness of CBASP for Hispanic/Latino clients. Finally, researchers should strive to examine whether a differential treatment will emerge within the many heterogeneous cultures that comprise the Hispanic/Latino population.

CHAPTER 3

The Assessment, Diagnosis, and Treatment of Psychiatric Disorders in African American Clients

Daniel L Hollar, Julia D Buckner, Jill M Holm-Denoma, Matthew C Waesche, LaRicka Wingate, and Michael D Anestis

Approximately 12% of United States citizens (33.9 million people) identify themselves as African American or black.[1] African American individuals are among the least likely people to seek and receive mental health care services. The percentage of African American individuals suffering from psychopathology that gets treatment is only half that of non-Hispanic European individuals.[2] In addition, non-Hispanic European clients are four to five times more likely than African American clients to return for continued mental health services after initially being treated.[3] Furthermore, African American individuals who do seek and receive treatment are more likely to use inpatient or emergency services, to be rehospitalized after inpatient services, and to be often admitted involuntarily to mental institutions than non-Hispanic European individuals.[4-6] According to the United States Surgeon General, African American clients often receive lower quality care, are less likely to seek help when they are in distress, and have less access to services than other Americans.[1]

What leads to these differences in health care utilization? It may be that variables such as bias, cultural attitudes, and socioeconomic status affect health care access for African American individuals. In this chapter, we will discuss the roles of client and clinician biases in mental health care, as well as how cultural attitudes may affect the provision and effectiveness of psychotherapy for African American individuals. In addition, we will outline social and economic factors that may promote or hinder therapy for this population. We will detail how each of these issues might play out clinically in the areas of assessment, diagnosis, and treatment through case examples from our community outpatient mental health facility as well as through a review of the existing empirical literature on the matter. When applicable, we will attempt to provide effective solutions to problems therapists and clients may face based on our collective clinical experience and in accordance with research findings. We will additionally provide a comprehensive case example to better illustrate how the therapy process with an African American client can be sensitively and competently conducted. Finally, we will provide suggestions for future research in the areas of assessment, diagnosis, and treatment of African American clients.

CLINICAL OBSERVATIONS
Assessment

Generally, assessment refers to the process of assigning objective information, in comparison with norms, to an individual or group to inform diagnosis and treatment. Factors that may affect the assessment of African American clients include biases among mental health professionals regarding African American people, a general mistrust of mental health professionals by some African American clients, a lack of understanding of the culture shared by many African American individuals, and socioeconomic factors.

Bias and mistrust in assessment of African American clients. During the assessment process, clinicians may gather data using standardized assessment instruments (e.g., intelligence tests and personality tests) that have been normed on largely European samples. Yet, it is often unknown whether such instruments are able to accurately assess African American clients. If they are not able to do so, the assessment may produce misleading information that may result in inaccurate diagnosis. There are many consequences to misdiagnosis, including the potential to cause clients to mistrust their mental health providers and/or the assessment process. Also, misdiagnosis can lead to inaccurate treatment recommendations. For reasons such as these, mental health practitioners should always make it a priority to use assessment instruments that are appropriate for use with African American clients.

What can clients and mental health care providers do to increase accurate assessment of African American clients? Clients and mental health care providers alike are encouraged to investigate whether the assessment tools being used have been normed on African American populations. Mental health care providers and clients may also want to determine if there are differences in interpretation guidelines for African American individuals.

To begin to address how clients' perceptions of bias influence assessment, it may be useful to first briefly discuss the origins of cultural mistrust in the history of psychological assessment of the African American community. Historically, many African American clients who sought health care services were misinformed, pathologized, overmedicated, given long-term and inpatient (rather than outpatient) treatment, and exposed to culturally insensitive clinicians.[7] Perhaps the most cited example of this trend is the Tuskegee Syphilis Study (1932–72). This study examined the treatment and course of syphilis in 400 African American sharecroppers. The researchers did not provide proper care to their participants. For instance, participants did not give informed consent and were not informed of their diagnosis. Rather, participants were told they had "bad blood" and not informed that they had a treatable sexually transmitted disease.[8] Consequences included the death of participants as well as the unknowing transmission of syphilis to others.

Sociological studies have shown that research experiments such as the Tuskegee Syphilis Study (e.g., see reference 9) have predisposed many African American individuals to distrust medical and public health authorities.[3] The Tuskegee Syphilis Study is likely to be a significant factor that contributes to the low number of African American participants in clinical trials as well as the underutilization of mental health services. Given that some African American clients may have developed a mistrust of the health care system generally and mental health care specifically, clinicians are also encouraged to assuage concerns clients may have about the assessment process. The following case example from our clinic illustrates ways in which client mistrust may be expressed clinically.

Tila, an African American client, presented to our clinic seeking a learning disorder assessment for her child. She openly expressed to the non-African American clinician an expectation that her child would be negatively evaluated if not assessed by an African American assessor. She also stated that she would more readily accept the results of the evaluation if the clinician were African American. When the clinician asked her to explain why she held this belief, Tila stated, "Everyone knows these tests are biased against blacks." She also reported that when she went to parent–teacher association meetings, many of the African American parents raised concern that their children could not pass the statewide-standardized tests because the tests were biased. Further, Tila indicated that she had taken some psychology courses in college and she recalled reading that all standardized IQ tests were culturally biased against African American individuals.

In situations such as these, we recommend that the clinician empathize with the client's concerns. Perhaps more importantly, the clinician should assure the parent that he or she would make every effort to use tests that have been evaluated for use with African American clients and to interpret the results in a manner that takes into account the cultural context in which assessment data are being collected (i.e., applying scientific mindedness, dynamic sizing, and culture-specific expertise[10]). The clinician should also provide psychoeducation to address the client's mistrust of non-African American therapists. For example, the clinician might employ culture-specific expertise through informing the client that research suggests that the race/ethnicity of the clinician does not necessarily result in biased interpretation of assessment scores (discussed below). In addition, utilizing scientific mindedness, the clinician can provide a list of clinics that may provide the same service should the client wish to seek a second opinion (i.e., testing the hypothesis) or a different clinician before accepting any conclusions about assessment data. Letting the client know they have control over the assessment process may help to allay any misconceived notions that the clinician has an ulterior or malicious motive during assessment.

It is important to openly discuss mistrust with clients when appropriate given that mistrust of mental health care professionals can affect the assessment process in several ways. Mistrust may lead some clients to withhold vital information necessary to a comprehensive assessment. The more open and honest a client is about life experiences, background, and symptom expression during assessment, the more informed a therapist can be to make an accurate diagnosis and select an appropriate treatment, referral, etc. Further, if mistrust occurs in one ethnic group more than in others, the potential for cultural bias in assessment becomes more likely because symptom expression may vary across ethnic groups. Therefore, the development of culturally sensitive assessment measures and the external validity of those measures are contingent on the openness and active participation of individuals from diverse ethnic groups.[11]

Mistrust of the health care system may also lead some clients to feel they need to control as many aspects of the therapeutic process as possible (perhaps to ensure they are not taken advantage of). Some clients may not seek mental health services unless they have some choice regarding the characteristics of the mental health professional with whom they will work. For instance, at times, clients seeking services at our community outpatient clinic make requests for a therapist of a particular race or gender. It is our clinic's policy to randomly assign clients to a therapist and it is rare to grant requests for a different therapist under most circumstances. There are several reasons for this approach. First, the clinic is a part of a state university's program for training clinical psychology graduate students and thus must provide equal opportunity for all its graduate student therapists to receive diverse training experiences. Second, clients are assigned on a first come, first served basis based on the availability of therapists to ensure each therapist has a full case load of clients and to minimize a client's time on the waiting list. Third, the clinic adheres to this policy to discourage clients from perpetuating any avoidant behaviors that may be contributing to the condition for which they may be seeking mental health services (e.g., many clients request a person of the same gender because they are seeking help for interpersonal problems with a person of the opposite gender). Finally, some research suggests that therapist race may not affect treatment outcome under certain conditions (discussed below). Therapists at our clinic are encouraged to provide rationale to clients about why their requests for a particular type of mental health care professional may not be honored, as rationale provision is known to help clients feel autonomous and competent.[12]

The role of cultural attitudes and beliefs in assessment. During the assessment process, culture-specific expertise of the cultural attitudes and beliefs to which a client may be oriented (e.g., an Africentric or European worldview) is necessary as it may possibly inform treatment objectives. Cultural attitudes and beliefs (i.e., worldview) can be described as the complex perspective one has concerning the nature of the universe, the nature of humankind, and the relation of these perspectives to philosophical issues that help us make sense of the world.[13] Cultural attitudes and beliefs represent an individual's social, political, and cultural orientation (e.g., an

African American may have a European orientation or an Africentric one), and are organized in a set of hypotheses and theories that an individual holds about the makeup of his or her world. Some examples of the Africentric worldview include: an emphasis on group and relationships, extended family structure, a focus on immediate and short range goals, and an indistinct view of mental and physical health.[14] Although every culture has its own set of attitudes and beliefs, it is important to note that there is also within-group variability, such that not all clients of the same ethnic or racial group will have the same worldview.[13]

Employing culture-specific expertise can improve assessment in many ways. For example, among some of our African American clients, descriptions of certain psychological symptoms of depression and anxiety are sometimes generally reported as "stress" or some other physical pain (e.g., headache, chest pains, and upset stomach), and this tendency makes it difficult to distinguish between the mental illness and physical maladies. Therapists should be aware of this cultural tendency for some African American individuals to report different types of emotional distress as somatic complaints.[15–17] A therapist, through dynamic sizing, must determine whether or not such tendencies exhibited by African American clients are accurate or the result of a cultural stereotype.

The following is a clinical example of how scientific mindedness, culture-specific expertise, and dynamic sizing can impact assessment. Jerry, a 34-year-old African American male client, sought services at our outpatient psychology clinic for feelings of depression and social isolation. As part of his assessment, Jerry completed the Minnesota Multiphasic Personality Inventory, Second Edition (MMPI-2).[18] The MMPI-2 is a self-report measure (normed on a primarily European sample) used to assess personality and clinical symptoms.[19] On interpretation, it was noted that Jerry elevated several clinical scales: scale 2 (which can be indicative of depressive symptomatology) and scale 8 (which can be indicative of feelings social and emotional isolation, unusual experiences, and/or sensory disturbances). This pattern of elevations may indicate the presence of severe psychopathology. In a display of scientific mindedness, the therapist questioned Jerry about why he endorsed certain critical items (e.g., those related to sensory disturbances) that may have contributed to the elevation of scale 8. Jerry explained that he had engaged in some criminal activity during adolescence (e.g., sold drugs, carried a handgun, joined a gang). He reported that at that time, he had many unusual and bizarre experiences (e.g., witnessed a murder, was shot, misused drugs and alcohol). Taking this information into consideration, in addition to considering other observations at the time of the interview (i.e., good interpersonal style, appropriate dress and grooming) the therapist concluded that the client's report was not indicative of psychotic symptomatology.

Socioeconomic factors relevant to the assessment of African American clients. Nearly a quarter of African American individuals earn more than US$50,000 a year, yet, when compared with other racial/ethnic groups in the United States, African American individuals continue to be relatively poor.[1] To illustrate, in 1999, approximately 22% of African American families lived in poverty, compared with 13% for the United States as a whole and 8% for non-Hispanic European individuals.[1] Because many African American people are of low socioeconomic status (SES) and therefore lack many financial resources, some of our African American clients have reported that they often rely on treatment strategies other than traditional mental health care facilities when experiencing psychological problems. For example, some African American clients treated at our clinic have reported that it is customary for their families to care for mentally ill loved ones at home. Those individuals who sought services outside the home reported they usually had first turned to extended family members, friends, or their church before seeking professional psychotherapeutic services. They often indicate that the primary reason for seeking therapeutic services from family, friends, church, etc., is that these services were free. Socioeconomic barriers such as lack of insurance, lack of transportation, and family responsibilities may also serve as barriers to mental health services for African American individuals.

African American individuals are less likely to seek treatment than non-African American groups.[1] The underutilization of mental health services not only affects those African American individuals who are ill and not receiving treatment, but it also limits the effectiveness of mental health services broadly. For instance, given that those clients who do seek services may not be representative of typical African American individuals, it may be harder for accurate assessment tools to be developed that can generalize to *all* individuals within the African American community. In addition, the lack of sufficient numbers of African American individuals available for assessment may also lead to inadequate training experiences for mental health care providers. The mental health community must therefore work to increase recruitment of African American clients by engaging in activities such as: raising awareness through outreach programs and advertisements at churches and community organization meetings, conducting advertising campaigns marketed toward African American individuals, and training therapists to be committed to delivering culturally sensitive services.[11,20–24]

Diagnosis

Diagnosis is the process of identifying pathology by its signs and symptoms using the results of various assessment procedures. The process of diagnostics can also be affected by bias among some mental health professionals, a mistrust of mental health professionals by some African American clients, and cultural barriers such as primarily relying on family and religious community during periods of distress.

Bias and cultural mistrust in diagnosis. Bias can affect the diagnostic process in several ways. For instance, given that the majority of the diagnostic criteria of the *Diagnostic and Statistical Manual of Mental Disorders* (DSM)[25] were developed using assessment data from largely European American samples, the criteria may be limited in their generalizability to minority populations.[24] It may also be the case that some clinicians may make diagnostic errors with African American clients due to clinician biases and a lack of understanding of African American culture.

Research indicates that it is common for people to hold some degree of stereotypic views of people of another race or social group.[26–28] Though many people may make efforts to control their own prejudice, mental health professionals are vulnerable to engaging in stereotyped thinking.[29] Some clinicians may hold stereotypic beliefs or make assumptions about their African American clients based on personal experiences or vicarious experiences such as images portrayed by the media (e.g., delinquent, unmotivated, nonintellectual, athletic, musical, humorous, etc.). Stereotypic views held by therapists may affect diagnoses in several ways. For example, a therapist could interpret a client's lack of employment as an indication of his or her laziness versus probing further to uncover that the client suffers from amotivation or anergia, both of which are symptoms of depression. Consistent with recommendations of the American Psychological Association (APA), we urge all mental health professionals to be aware of their own biases or stereotypic views before entering into a therapeutic relationship with a person from another culture.[30] Being mindful of one's own beliefs and biases (i.e., scientific mindedness[10]) can minimize the application of stereotypic beliefs to diagnostic decisions. When clinicians have not been scientific minded, research shows that African American clients end up with higher rates of diagnosed schizophrenia than expected compared with European American clients.[31]

The role of cultural attitudes and beliefs in diagnosis. Cultural norms for what constitute "abnormal" behavior may be different for African American individuals than for non-African American groups. Some African American people may have different ways of expressing symptoms and complaints, exhibit different culturally normative behaviors, and display different coping mechanisms than some European individuals. For example, some African American clients in our clinic have endorsed beliefs such as "someone is conspiring against me" or "people are talking about me." When working with a client who has such beliefs, a clinician should consider a diagnosis of paranoid personality disorder or a schizophrenia-spectrum disorder. Yet, when working with minority clients, therapists should also consider the possibly that experiences of racism may account for seemingly paranoid beliefs among members of minority groups. For instance, one client at our clinic reported suspicious feelings that people were always talking badly about him. On further questioning, he reported the reason he believed people were talking malevolently about him was that he was the only African American man in his work environment and that his past experiences in similar situations had resulted in out-group member discrimination. Given this information, the therapist must consider the possibility that this client was not paranoid but was rather reporting a legitimate observation.

Treatment

Treatment refers to the application of appropriate psychological services according to assessment and diagnostic findings. In this chapter, treatment will refer to the use of empirically supported psychotherapies (i.e., those treatments that have demonstrated research-based efficacy or effectiveness for a particular disorder).[32]

Mental health professional bias in treatment of African American individuals. There are times when a mental health professional's personal bias or beliefs may interfere with the treatment of some clients. For example, if the clinician adheres to the stereotype that African American individuals are lazier than other groups, that clinician may believe that African American clients will not adhere to treatment protocols. Such biased clinicians may therefore behave in a manner toward African American clients that discourages them from pursuing mental health services (e.g., be less likely to work to increase motivation on treatment noncompliance). Similarly, African American clients who believe treatment cannot be delivered by non-African American therapists may also encounter limited treatment options, especially in areas where the number of African American therapists is limited. It is therefore necessary for mental health care professionals to educate clinicians, researchers, and community members alike about the dangers of stereotypes and bias in the delivery and perceptions of mental health services.

The role of cultural attitudes and beliefs in treatment. A broad array of cultural factors plays a role in how African American clients respond to psychiatric care. An individual's beliefs and expectations about treatment may determine adherence to and the success of psychotherapy. For instance, there appears to be a belief in the African American community against the prolonged use of prescription medications. At our clinic, some African American clients have expressed distrust of the addictive potential of medications and the associated negative stigma of addiction. To illustrate, some African American clients have reported extreme concern that they will become addicted to medications such as alprazolam (Xanax) or methylphenidate (Ritalin). Given that some medications do exhibit increased addiction potential (e.g., alprazolam[33]) whereas others do not, we recommend psychoeducation about the each medication's addictive properties and the importance of adhering to prescription instructions. We also recommend encouraging clients to express concerns to their medical doctors, as well as providing psychoeducation on alternatives to medication interventions when appropriate (e.g., psychotherapy). Given the hesitation of some African American clients to use prescription medication, clinicians and psychiatrists may want to ask whether patients are using alternative or herbal therapies (as may sometimes be the case in this population; see reference 34). Overlooking possible interactions and side effects of the drugs and herbal remedies may make it more likely that African American clients will discontinue psychotropics, thereby potentially limiting treatment gains.

To illustrate issues related to medication adherence in this population: one of our African American clients, Diamond, was being treated with cognitive-behavioral therapy (CBT)[35] for depression while also taking Ritalin for attention deficit hyperactivity disorder (ADHD). During the course of treatment, it became increasingly difficult to conduct the CBT tasks in session. The therapist asked Diamond about her medication adherence. Diamond replied that she did not want to take her medication anymore, so her mother allowed her to try a semester off medication. Diamond's mother reported that her decision was in part due to negative publicity Ritalin was getting from people in the community and in the media. During her time off of the medication, Diamond had great difficulty concentrating, listening, paying attention, following directions, and was inconsistent with her schoolwork, often not trying more difficult assignments. The therapist explained that other medications were available (e.g., Listol and atomoxetine [Strattera]) and outlined to Diamond's mother how the lack of medication was affecting therapy. After psychoeducation on the combined effects of psychotherapy and medication, Diamond resumed medication (as prescribed by her physician) and demonstrated subsequent treatment gains.

Spirituality serves as another important cultural factor in the lives of many African American individuals. As discussed above, many African American individuals turn to the church when dealing with mental and physical health issues.[36] It is possible that the African American individuals who break with this cultural norm of church utilization and seek psychological services outside the church may be suffering from more severe symptomatology (i.e., longer duration or recurrence of problematic behaviors), and thus more difficult to treat. When treating African American individuals, it may be important to assess religious/ spiritual involvement for several reasons. Church membership may be a protective factor and a good prognostic indicator for treatment. Discontinuation of church attendance could be an indicator of degree of functional impairment and may provide temporal information regarding the onset of depressive symptomatology such as anhedonia. When treating African American clients, it may be useful to suggest church involvement (if consistent with the client's personal religious/ spiritual beliefs) as a source of social support and behavioral activation.

Socioeconomic factors in the treatment of African American clients. As discussed above, African American individuals are overrepresented in the low SES group.[37] Thus, cost may serve as a significant barrier to treatment for many African American clients. Although our clinic operates on a sliding scale, many African American clients request additional fee reductions because they cannot afford the extra expenditure for therapy. Lack of available funds affects treatment effectiveness because many clients cannot commit to weekly visits despite psychoeducation regarding the decreased effectiveness of reduced frequency of sessions.

Some low SES clients do not own their own vehicles and depend on either public transportation or friends to take them to the clinic. Thus, lack of transportation may affect treatment as well. To address these treatment barriers, clinicians are encouraged to be creative in devising ways to accommodate their clients (e.g., giving clients weekly homework assignments even though they may only be able to attend treatment on a monthly basis, employing Motivational Interviewing (MI)[38] to enhance commitment to therapy, considering phone therapy sessions if transportation is a problem, using psychoeducation to emphasize the importance of consistent, weekly psychotherapy).

THE CURRENT STATE OF THE LITERATURE

The extant empirical literature supports the assertion that the assessment, diagnosis, and treatment of African American clients may be complicated by cultural issues. In this section, we will outline the emerging data concerning culturally competent delivery of mental health services for African American clients.

Assessment

There has been wide debate over racial biases in different forms of assessment (e.g., intelligence tests, standardized symptom inventories). One assessment that has been at the center of this discussion is the widely used MMPI-2. Developed to assess psychological symptomatology and personality characteristics, the MMPI-2 has become an important tool in many mental health assessments. Although the MMPI-2 certainly provides diagnostically relevant information, questions about its ability to accurately assess African American clients have arisen.

One facet of the MMPI-2 that makes it particularly attractive to mental health professionals is its well-developed battery of validity scales, which help to identify individuals attempting to falsify or misrepresent themselves on the test. Research has suggested that small, but consistent differences exist in the test's F scale (Infrequency), which measures possible malingering or exaggeration of symptoms, for African American individuals when compared with Europeans.[39-41] Further, African American people have been shown to exhibit elevations on scales 8 (schizophrenia) and 9 (hypomania) of the MMPI-2 when compared with European individuals.[39-41] These scales are used to assess and infer severe psychopathology. Such elevations could lead test interpreters to incorrectly conclude that an African American individual is more psychologically disturbed or distressed than is actually the case.

At present, there appear to at least be two main explanations for the differences between African American and European clients on the MMPI-2. The first explanation involves SES. Research has consistently found that the differential elevations found on African American clients' MMPI-2 scales are attenuated or disappear completely once one controls for demographic variables such as income and education.[42] In other words, the differences seen in the scores of African American people may, in fact, be mediated by income and education. Further, differential life experiences and an Africentric worldview may account for the disparities between races in assessment scales.[40] Higher scores observed on these scales in many African American samples have been interpreted by some to be indicative of cultural differences in perception and expectations, rather than pathology.[43] Thus, clinicians are urged to incorporate scientifically derived information, such as racial and SES differences in MMPI-2 scores, when interpreting their client's assessment results.

In addition to personality inventories such as the MMPI-2, clinicians are often called upon to administer tests that measure intelligence (also called intelligence quotient or "IQ"). According to Eysenck,[44] IQ is an individual's obtained score relative to that of his or her peer group, based on a group of standardized tests devised to assess different cognitive abilities. As with the MMPI-2, the use of IQ tests with African American clients has been questioned.[45,46] For instance, African

American and Latino individuals have scored, on average, 12–15 points lower than European individuals on IQ tests.[47]

One explanation for observed differences in IQ scores between European and African American individuals is that different scores are the result of different cultural beliefs and/or historical experiences (e.g., victimization, racism, oppression, prejudice, discrimination, miseducation, dependence, poverty). For example, when African American individuals experience racism, the acculturative stress is significant enough to be both physically and psychologically debilitating to the health of that individual.[48] In addition, having experienced approximately 400 years of slavery and oppression, African American individuals may have formed adaptive problem-solving styles that are inherently different from individuals who have not had that experience. In accordance with scientific mindedness, future research is warranted to examine this hypothesis or other possible explanations.

Diagnosis

Accurately diagnosing mental illness can be difficult, but is nevertheless a vital task for any mental health practitioner, as diagnosis informs appropriate treatment. Evidence suggests that African American clients are more vulnerable to certain types of misdiagnosis than are European individuals.[31,49–54] As discussed below, the reasons for these misdiagnoses are complex.

Research indicates that some disorders may be underdiagnosed in the African American community, whereas others are overdiagnosed. For example, European adults with depression or anxiety disorders are more likely to receive treatment than African American adults with the same disorders, even though the disorders occur in both groups at about the same rate after controlling for differences in SES.[1] Data from primary care and emergency room settings suggest that African American clients are accurately diagnosed with depression less often than European clients.[49,54] In addition, African American patients present with disproportionately high rates of schizophrenia and disproportionately low rates of affective disorders.[31] Further, psychotic symptomatology (a characteristic of several distinct mental disorders) is more likely to lead mental health professionals to diagnose bipolar disorder in European clients and schizophrenia in African American clients.[55–57] African American youths have been diagnosed as having mental retardation or placed in special education programs at higher than expected rates.[50–53] African American clients are more likely to be diagnosed with antisocial personality disorder or paranoid personality disorder relative to European patients,[58] although the symptoms clinicians may observe that point to these diagnoses may be more indicative of unique experiences that African American individuals have rather than true personality pathology.

There are, however, some illnesses for which African American individuals experience what appear to be legitimately lower base rates. Most notably among these are eating disorders.[59] While awareness of lower base rates is useful to prevent overdiagnosis, it is important that mental health professionals be mindful of individual differences among the individuals who comprise the African American community and not minimalize eating disorder symptomatology in African American girls with an eating disorder.[59] Similarly, African American individuals complete suicide at lower rates than European individuals.[60,61] Again, it is important for clinicians to not overlook indicators of potential suicidal behavior in African American individuals who are genuinely experiencing suicidal symptoms.

The diagnosis of mental illness in African American clients is complicated by findings that the same mental illness might be manifested by different symptoms in African American clients than in European clients. African American individuals who have major depressive disorder (MDD), for example, are more likely to present with sleep disturbance and appetite change than European individuals with MDD.[62] Further, African American clients with MDD report less pessimism, self-blame, and suicidal ideation than European individuals with MDD.[62] These differential symptoms patterns could lead to inaccurate diagnosis if the diagnostician is unaware of these differences.

Treatment

Despite clinical observations that treatment may be affected by the cultural factors discussed above, research on treatment for African American clients is generally lacking. The scarce research that exists divides its focus into two key areas: (i) the debate whether African American clients benefit from client–therapist racial matching and (ii) current findings on the effectiveness and efficacy of various treatment modules that were developed primarily among European individuals and yet are frequently applied to African American clients. Additional research is needed to further clarify these issues, but an examination of current findings will serve to reveal several robust findings and promising results.

The data have been mixed regarding the benefits of racial matching of client and therapist.[63-65] In addition, results have been equivocal with regard to African American clients' level of preference for racially similar therapists. Although some African American clients prefer African American therapists,[66] there is evidence suggesting that even when racial similarity is preferred, African American clients consider it less important than characteristics of therapist competency (education, personality, attitudes).[67] Thus, even when present, racial/ethnic preference is secondary in importance to other therapist characteristics and may not have as large an impact on treatment attrition as other therapist characteristics.

Patient preference for racial/ethnic similarity, however, is not the only variable that may influence whether client–therapist race matching is more effective than nonmatched racial pairings. An additional question to consider is whether therapist–client racial matching affects attrition. Currently, the evidence is equivocal, as conflicting results have emerged regarding whether racial/ethnic matching affects client drop-out rates.[10,68] Furthermore, it is important to consider if ethnically relevant variables such as language and acculturation level may moderate the importance of client–therapist racial matching. In other minority populations, moderator variables have been identified. For instance, among Mexican American clients, Global Assessment of Functioning (GAF) scores at termination were related to race matching among clients for whom Spanish was their main language.[69] Thus, it is possible that among certain groups of African American clients (e.g., those who strongly relate to an Africentric worldview or those who have not acculturated to mainstream European culture), certain variables may moderate the general conclusions about the relative unimportance of therapist–client racial matching. Unfortunately, there is currently a paucity of research examining issues such as these among African American clients.

Regardless of the racial or ethnic background of the therapist, empirically supported treatments for particular disorders appear to be effective for African American clients. CBT is effective in treating African American clients with minor depression (defined in the DSM-IV-TR appendix as a mood disturbance featuring at least two but less than five symptoms of MDD over the period of two weeks or more[25,70]). Interpersonal Psychotherapy (IPT)[71] also appears an effective treatment for depression among African American patients.[72] However, higher attrition rates have been observed for African American patients than for European patients with regard to this treatment modality, with a significantly higher proportion of African American clients failing to complete the continuation phase of IPT.[72] Although additional research is necessary to determine the reasons for the higher attrition rates, the success of empirically supported treatments for depressive disorders among African American patients is a significant and promising finding.

Treatment outcome studies for African American clients with anxiety disorders have been more limited. CBT has been found to be equally effective in reducing anxiety symptoms (as measured by both teacher and parent reports) for African American and European children with anxiety disorders.[42] In a case study of two African American adults, behavioral treatment was effective for the treatment of obsessive-compulsive disorder.[73] This limited research suggests that CBT for anxiety may be effective for African American clients.

Promising results have also been found in studies on treatment outcome for African American clients with chronic mental illness and comorbid psychotic and substance use disorders (SUDs). In one study, a significant level of improvement was sustained over the course of a two-year follow-up in a sample of 32 African American patients with chronic mental illness (e.g. schizophrenia, mood disorders). In addition, the four patients with comorbid psychotic disorder and SUD improved significantly.[74] Similarly promising, community-based psychosocial rehabilitation programs have resulted in positive outcomes for African American clients with schizophrenia, as measured by clinical change, functional change, and subjective experience change.[62] The rate of overall improvement in these clients was slower than that of European clients, but the end results were the same, indicating that the treatment itself is effective. In these studies, the one area in which African American clients showed significantly less improvement was social functioning.[74] Additional research in this area would be invaluable to uncover factors that contribute to these decreased levels of post-treatment social functioning.

Additional research is necessary to improve the assessment, diagnosis, and treatment of African American clients. Longitudinal research on empirically supported treatment outcomes for African American clients is needed to more fully understand whether current treatments are effective with this population. Further research is also necessary to determine what factors may contribute to lower social functioning and higher attrition rates among African American clients relative to other clients. Clarification of these issues will allow for increases in the overall quality of mental health care for a significant portion of the population.

COMPREHENSIVE CASE ILLUSTRATION

The following case example strives to illustrate a culturally competent approach (i.e., culture-specific expertise, dynamic sizing, and scientific mindedness) to the delivery of mental health services for African American clients, consistent with the empirical and clinical data discussed above.

Troy was a 30-year-old, single African American man who worked as a customer service representative for a temporary agency. Troy's general physician referred Troy to our clinic due to his complaints of constant stress, irritability, and back pain. During his initial visit, Troy stated that he had a lack of desire to socialize with friends and family, and often experienced problems with irritability and concentration. He had a 10-year-old son who lived with the boy's mother in Washington, DC. Troy described his relationship with his son as "very good" and stated that he was more "emotional" with his son than with other people. He reported that he was currently involved in a romantic relationship. Troy indicated that he was unsure about participating in therapy, stating that he was "not crazy." In addition, he reported that he did not have insurance and could not afford the cost of therapy.

Troy was born and raised (primarily by his grandmother) in an urban area of Washington, DC. He never had a relationship with his father and reported no relationship with his mother since he was 11 years old. He stated that his mother misused cocaine and neglected him when he was a child. Troy denied difficulties with depression, anxiety, or substance use, and reported good eating habits. Troy stated that he thought his problems with concentration and stress were "holding back" his progress in life. He reported that he often had nightmares of events he had experienced in his past (e.g., being shot at, seeing friends get shot, seeing people die).

Troy completed a structured clinical interview as well as several self-report measures designed to assess his emotional state and behavioral functioning, which included the Beck Suicide Scale (BSS),[75] Beck Anxiety Inventory (BAI),[76] and the Beck Depression Inventory (BDI).[77] Although Troy did not report any significant problems with anxiety (BAI total=5) or suicidality (BSS=0), his overall score on the BDI (17) was indicative of the presence of some depressive symptoms. Troy's MMPI-2 scores were elevated on scales 8 (schizophrenia, T score=75) and 4 (psychopathic deviate, T score=68). It is important to note that elevations on both scales 8 and 4 are often consistent with individuals who may not fit into society very well and who are often seen as nonconforming, angry, and irritable. Typically, people with this profile are socially isolated and avoid close relationships. These elevations often indicate resentment toward authority, distrust of others, and involvement in criminal acts.

Troy's therapist approached the interpretation of Troy's assessment data with scientific mindedness. For instance, the therapist was mindful that African American clients sometimes display a higher elevation of scale 8 on the MMPI-2, and took care to probe Troy's specific item responses for cultural variation in endorsement of particular items. As Troy explained why he endorsed particular items, it became clear the elevation of scale 8 was the result of particular life experiences (e.g., being shot at, seeing friends get shot, seeing people die).

As Troy expressed ambivalence about the prospect of therapy, the therapist thoroughly discussed and responded to Troy's concerns.

> *Therapist*: Through different experiences in our lives, such as watching TV and movies, talking with friends and family, and watching others, we all tend to develop some picture in our minds of what therapy is. Will you tell me about the idea of therapy that you have in your mind? There is no right or wrong answer.

> *Troy*: I don't know anybody who has gone to therapy. I guess I always thought therapy was for crazy people. Now, I know some crazy people, but I just see them on the streets, I don't think they go to therapy. Growing up, when my mom had nerves, was stressed, or was sad, she went to talk to her pastor.

The therapist empathized with Troy's concerns and provided psychoeducation about the nature of therapy (e.g., a person does not have to be "crazy" to attend therapy, the benefits of treatment for Troy's stress and related back pain). To be sensitive to the possible financial obstacle, the therapist secured Troy a reduced fee for therapy. Troy chose to participate in psychotherapy because he felt the therapist "tried to understand and help" him.

Troy participated in individual therapy to explore the issues related to his expressed symptomatology, as well as ongoing difficulties related to his early life experiences. Given Troy's depressive symptomatology and interpersonal difficulties, Cognitive Behavioral Analysis System of Psychotherapy (CBASP)[78] was determined to be the treatment of choice for Troy. This approach asked Troy to analyze recent, specific situations that occurred in his life. The therapist encouraged the client to define the situation, as well as the actual and desired outcomes of that situation. Together, therapist and client examined the actual thoughts and behaviors the client had during the situation. They then worked together to adjust those thoughts and behaviors in a way that would better achieve the client's desired outcome. Troy responded well to CBASP, reporting that he had began to think more about how he could influence the situations he was in as well as his mood. Once he learned that he could influence his mood and situations with simple behaviors and changing his thought patterns, his mood increased and his stress significantly decreased, as indicated by both standardized measures and self-report. He once stated, "I feel like a king. I didn't know I had so much power." Troy reported that he no longer felt back pain and that he was more able to open up to people and had made several new and trusted friends since beginning therapy.

It is important to note that the therapist and client in the above illustration were of the same race, which may have assisted in the building of rapport and the client's willingness to commit to the therapeutic process. Thus, it appears the initial barrier to treatment was the client's beliefs about the process of therapy itself and not the therapist's race. However, if race would have been a barrier, we believe that through employing the same procedures of culture-specific expertise, dynamic sizing, and scientific mindedness the clinician could allay that concern as well. For example, through psychoeducation about clinician–client matching and treatment effectiveness, discussion of cultural barriers and stereotypes, or the clinician's acknowledgment of limited experience with the client's history of oppression, a therapist could strengthen rapport and increase the client's commitment to the therapeutic process.

CONCLUSIONS AND FUTURE DIRECTIONS

Empirical research regarding clinical work with African American clients is lacking in several domains. Given that African American individuals are less likely to seek out mental health services than members of other racial groups, our current understanding of the generalizability of current mental health practices to these clients is limited. Research is necessary to address a number of questions, including whether African American individuals experience prejudice in therapy and how stereotypes and bias affect clinician–client interactions. In addition, the generalizability of current assessment instruments and current diagnostic criteria need to be established.

Given differential treatment attrition rates, it is also necessary for future research to investigate ways to increase treatment compliance among African American clients. Further, although emerging data suggest that empirically supported treatments are equally effective for African American clients as for European clients, this finding has not been replicated for all empirical treatments. For instance, there is good reason to believe CBASP will be effective for African American clients (as discussed above). Research is also needed to determine whether there are changes that could be made to standard protocols to provide even better help to African American clients.

In addition to the need for empirical studies, psychoeducation needs to be provided to therapists regarding the treatment of African American clients.[30] Consistent with APA guidelines, psychoeducation on the experiences of African American people should be provided as part of training programs and continuing education. It is also important for therapists to identify their particular views and biases, and make efforts to reduce their biases from interfering with treatment through available methods (e.g., continuing education, consultation, education).

Morris[13] provided a number of suggestions for working with clients of an African American background. First, assessment must take into consideration how the client identifies him or herself (i.e., African American) as well as the extent to which they participate in the cultural traditions of the majority culture. Assessment and the appropriateness of a diagnosis and treatment are contingent on these factors. For instance, if it is a normal and nondistressing part of a client's religion to hear voices speaking to them and to believe that they are on a special mission from God, these may not be considered symptoms of psychopathology. However, if the client fully participates in the traditions of mainstream society and is therefore distressed or impaired by voices, etc., these same acts may be considered pathological. In addition, Morris suggested that therapists be willing to adopt flexible roles, be sensitive to cultural idiosyncrasies, and be willing to discuss racial differences. Therapists should also include questions about church activity and extended family relationships in the assessment and therapy process, use problem-solving therapies that focus on a client's everyday experiences and strengths (rather than on deficits), and use the client's cultural contexts as the foundation for diagnostic clarification and inquiry. It is of note that Morris's suggestions are not only applicable to working with African American clients, but also to clients from any background.

Based on clinical experience and a thorough review of relevant literature, the importance of including the client's cultural context in the assessment, diagnosis, and treatment of African American clients has been illustrated above. Clinically, African American people who are distressed or have a mental illness may present their symptoms according to certain norms in their cultural group. This may lead to misdiagnosis if the symptom profiles differ from what the mental health professional has been trained to assess. The treatments that we use at our community-based clinic have been empirically supported and use nonvalue-based therapies (i.e., CBT, CBASP, MI), which should be effective in diverse ethnic groups, although research is needed to evaluate this hypothesis. Current research suggests that the assessment, diagnosis, and treatment of African American clients may be complicated by biases or miscomprehension on the part of mental health practitioners, clients' beliefs that non-African American therapists may not be able to understand them, instrument bias, and cultural phenomena that are unique to African American individuals. These factors illustrate the need for culturally competent assessment, diagnosis, and treatment. In the meantime, culture-specific expertise, dynamic sizing, and scientific mindedness are provisions clinicians can use to assist in the overall quality of mental health care for a significant portion of African American clients.

CHAPTER 4

The Assessment, Diagnosis, and Treatment of Psychiatric Disorders in Lesbian, Gay, and Bisexual Clients

Kathryn H Gordon, and Yezzennya Castro

Estimates of the prevalence of lesbian, gay, and bisexual (LGB) individuals in the general population have varied from 2% to 10%.[1-3] Moreover, it has been estimated that LGB individuals utilize therapy at higher rates than individuals who are not of minority sexual orientation status,[4,5] and that most therapists report seeing at least one LGB client in their practice.[6] Therefore, it is of the utmost importance that clinicians know how to appropriately provide mental health services for this population. This is particularly important in light of the past prejudicial treatment of LGB individuals by some mental health organizations.

The historical conceptualization of homosexuality as a mental disorder by the major associations of psychology and psychiatry is one clear example of cultural insensitivity toward LGB individuals by people in the field of mental health. Homosexuality was included as a mental illness in the original *Diagnostic and Statistical Manual of Mental Disorders* (DSM)[7] under "sociopathic personality disorders". Interestingly, sociopathic personality disorders were characterized by the absence of distress despite the presence of profound pathology. This meant that, while the current definition of a mental illness requires the experience of distress, the original DSM defined mental illness by the mere presence of a particular behavior. As such, homosexual men and women could still be labeled as mentally disordered even in the absence of significant distress or functional impairment.

Furthermore, the societal view of sexual behavior at the time was that appropriate sexual behavior was limited to only that which could potentially lead to procreation. In the DSM-II,[8] homosexuality as a mental illness was moved to "Sexual Deviations". The DSM-II stated that this category included "sexual interests that are directed primarily toward objects other than people of the opposite sex . . ." (p. 44) and also included the diagnoses of pedophilia, exhibitionism, voyeurism, sadism, and masochism. Therefore, the decision to classify homosexuality a mental illness could be conceptualized as a deficit model of mental illness: that is, a minority group was compared with the majority and where differences existed, that minority group was labeled as disordered, despite lack of evidence that this group was impaired or distressed by their sexual orientation.

In 1973, largely due to the arguments made by gay rights activists (backed by empirical data, e.g., Hooker[9]), the American Psychiatric Association removed homosexuality from its list of mental disorders. It has been over 30 years since homosexuality has been considered a mental disorder, but some mental health professionals continue to practice as though homosexuality and bisexuality constitute mental illnesses. For example, some practitioners still advertise therapeutic cures for homosexuality – usually called reparative or sexual reorientation therapy. Sexual reorientation therapy continues to be practiced by some clinicians,[10] despite the fact that the American Psychological Association (APA) and the American Psychiatric Association have both banned its administration. Reviews of the existing research on sexual reorientation therapy have found that it is not only largely ineffective at changing one's sexual orientation from homosexual to heterosexual, but that it is also connected to some harmful effects on the individual's mental health, such as depression, interpersonal difficulties, internalized homophobia, and suicidal ideation.[5,11–13] The continued practice of sexual orientation therapy by some therapists serves to maintain the notion that homosexuality is a mental illness, and may make LGB individuals hesitant to seek services.

There are mixed data on the base rates of psychiatric disorders in LGB individuals as compared with heterosexual individuals. In some studies there were no significant differences in psychological functioning between groups,[14,15] whereas others found that there were higher rates of mental illness among LGB individuals.[4,16] If LGB individuals are at greater risk for mental disorders, it may be due to factors such as less access to appropriate psychological services or the societal stigma that is associated with having a homosexual or bisexual sexual orientation. The potential heightened risk for mental illness among LGB individuals, therefore, is not to be considered a direct result of one's sexual orientation. Rather, an LGB person's increased experiences with stressors such as discrimination, violence, and prejudice may lead to the development of mental health problems such as mood, anxiety, or substance use disorders. This hypothesis is supported by data that demonstrate a reduction in the disparity between psychological distress in homosexual/bisexual individuals and heterosexual individuals after experience of discrimination is statistically controlled.[17]

In 2000, the APA published guidelines for psychotherapy with LGB clients,[18] in an effort "to provide practitioners with (1) a frame of reference for the treatment of lesbian, gay, and bisexual clients, and (2) basic information and further references in the areas of assessment, intervention, identity, relationships, and the education and training of psychologists." The guidelines note that the APA's 1975 statement, "Homosexuality per se implies no impairment in judgment, stability, reliability, or general social or vocational capabilities . . . and mental health professionals should take the lead in removing the stigma of mental illness long associated with homosexual orientation" was the beginning of a movement to make the field of mental health more accommodating to LGB clients' needs. However, there are still areas where psychologists are responsible for ensuring that their practice reflects the meaning of this statement. The guidelines identify important areas of consideration for psychologists who work with LGB clients, and also provide resources on the subject matter.

The APA guidelines describe special considerations for assessment, diagnosis, and treatment of mental illness in LGB clients.[18] The first section specifically describes the viewpoint that clinicians are encouraged to have on bisexuality and homosexuality in terms of their practice. First of all, psychologists should understand that homosexuality and bisexuality do not serve as makers of mental illness. That is, even if a client's stressors are related to their sexuality (e.g., discrimination), it is the *discrimination* that is responsible for the distress, not an individual's sexual orientation. In addition, psychologists are encouraged to take time to evaluate their personal views of homosexuality and bisexuality, and determine if their views could impede proper assessment and treatment of LGB individuals. This is where use of dynamic sizing, the therapist's ability to appropriately apply knowledge of the client's background and be aware of how their own biases affect therapy,[19] is necessary for delivery of culturally sensitive services. Clinicians are also urged to develop culture-specific expertise,[19] so that their views of homosexuality and bisexuality are informed by facts. If, after taking these steps to identify one's views and educate oneself with the facts about homosexuality and bisexuality, clinicians cannot divorce their personal views (if different) from the APA's views in practice, they are encouraged to refer their clients elsewhere. This will minimize the chances that LGB clients receive irresponsible or unethical psychological services. Finally, psychologists should strive to understand how inaccurate or prejudicial views of homosexuality and bisexuality, including their own, can propagate harmful stereotypes. Psychologists should be careful to not attribute mental health problems to homosexuality or bisexuality; rather, the problems should be attributed to the correlates associated with LGB individuals (e.g., more likely to be violently attacked, discriminated against).[20] Therapists who utilize a scientific mindedness approach (i.e. use the scientific method to investigate one's ideas of how the client's culture may affect assessment, diagnosis and/or treatment)[19] to their treatment of mental disorders in LGB clients will be less susceptible to proliferate harmful views of LGB individuals.

Other areas to be considered when working with LGB clients include family structure differences and diversity within the LGB population. It may be the case that LGB clients more often have family members who are not legally or biologically related to them. In addition, they may have issues related to their family of origin's acceptance or rejection of their sexual orientation. Psychologists are urged to respect these differences and educate themselves about what these family issues might mean by reading resources that are available for working with LGB clients.[21]

Clinicians should also respect differences within the LGB population. Cultures vary in their views of homosexuality and bisexuality, and it is important to be aware of how such differences can impact the client. The client should serve as the ultimate resource for describing the impact their ethnicity, age, religious views, etc. have on their view of themselves and their experience as an LGB person. Thus, clinicians are encouraged to place the client's behavior in the proper cultural context and ask clients about how these factors might affect them, rather than making assumptions about the client based on stereotypes.[5]

It is also recommended that psychologists put forth an effort to inform themselves about the above issues through reading scientific literature and also by directly asking the client about how these issues may or may not relate to their own experience. The main points of the APA's guidelines[18] can be summarized into three statements:

- Psychologists should not consider homosexuality or bisexuality to be a marker of mental illness

- Psychologists should not attribute distress or impairment to the client's sexuality, but rather the experiences that are often correlated with homosexuality and bisexuality

- Psychologists are responsible for educating themselves on common LGB issues, as well as making themselves aware of individual differences within LGB individuals.

This chapter aims to explain how the important LGB issues mentioned above can be integrated and considered while utilizing empirically supported treatments in LGB clients. First, we will discuss our clinical experiences and hypotheses regarding the assessment, diagnostics, and treatment of mental illness in LGB clients. Second, we will review the existing literature on assessment, diagnostics, and treatment in LGB clients. Third, we will present a case example that ties together our hypotheses with the research literature in the area. Finally, we will conclude and identify avenues for future research. We want to emphasize that we believe that most empirically supported treatments require little, if any, adjustment to be effective with LGB clients because most therapeutic interventions affect basic human processes that exist across people of diverse sexual orientations. Education about LGB issues is important for assessment, diagnosis (specifically, determining if their behavior is normal within cultural norms), and mental health treatment in LGB clients as discussed below.

This chapter focuses on how to adapt treatment in light of these special considerations, and also highlights instances in which treatment does not need to be adapted. Most of the adaptation of treatment concerns the therapist being educated in and aware of particular issues that LGB clients face and potential therapist bias toward LGB clients that may interfere with proper service delivery. Adaptation may also include focus on themes in therapy that may be more common among LGB clients (e.g., sexual identity, impact on family of origin, discrimination). Again, the general *framework* (or *process*) of empirically supported treatments probably does not require much adaptation, but the *content* may be different.

CLINICAL OBSERVATIONS

Assessment

The following section will discuss assessment issues during intake and throughout treatment (e.g., symptom change during treatment). In our clinical experience, the assessment process with LGB clients is quite similar to the assessment process with heterosexual clients. However, there may be a higher likelihood that sexual identity concerns will arise either at the beginning or during the course of therapy. Still, it should not be assumed that these concerns will necessarily be part of therapy with LGB clients – as these clients may be presenting for the treatment of a mental disorder unrelated to their experiences as a LGB individual. For example, a female client presented at our outpatient clinic with bipolar disorder. She, like two-thirds of LGB clients in one survey,[22] viewed her problems as having nothing to do with her sexual orientation. Therefore, the assessment process included virtually no discussion of her sexual orientation. She would mention her relationships with females as content in the therapeutic process, but the empirically supported treatment she received for bipolar disorder (social rhythms therapy[23] as adjunctive to antimanic medicines) required no adaptation.

However, when sexual identity issues do come up in therapy, it is important to assess what it is about the sexual identity that is distressing to the client. For instance, one client initially presented with anger problems, but issues about his sexuality arose as therapy progressed. He then wished to devote some time in therapy to his feelings of uncertainty about his sexuality, and distress about the fact that he might be homosexual. Regardless of the presenting problem, it is important for the clinician to consider that prejudice (e.g., stigma or family/friend reaction) may be the cause rather than the individual's sexual orientation. To illustrate, the aforementioned client was not distressed because of his homosexuality, but rather, the implications that he believed came along with being homosexual. For example, this client feared that if he were homosexual, he could not have the family he always wanted or be a successful business person.

Even when sexuality issues are not what prompt an LGB client to seek psychological services, therapists should not be blind to the unique experiences of homosexual and bisexual individuals when conceptualizing cases. Additionally, therapists should feel comfortable talking about same-sex relationships. Some clients may be attuned to even seemingly subtle avoidances of talking about same-sex relationships including: changing the topic, talking around the issue (rather than using plain sexual terms), or physical signs of discomfort (e.g., avoiding eye contact). In the same vein, therapists should not assume that their client is heterosexual. This assumption can manifest clinically in a scenario where the therapist is inquiring about romantic relationships and assumes that the romantic partner is of opposite sex. Therapists should strive to ask questions that do not assume sexual orientation, such as, "Has a *significant other* ever had a problem with your drinking habits?" rather than asking, "Has a *girlfriend* ever had problems with your drinking habits?"

In our clinical experience with the assessment of LGB clients, the standardized measures that are typically used with heterosexual clients can still be utilized. Again, when the clinician is interpreting the results, it is particularly important for the mental health symptoms (e.g., depression, anxiety, etc.) to not be attributed to the sexual orientation of the person. Rather, the clinician should take a scientific-minded approach and formulate hypotheses, as with any client, as to the sources of the distress. The therapist should then look for evidence in support of or against the hypotheses. The mental health symptoms may have nothing to do with events surrounding the sexual orientation of the individual, and practitioners should guard against such assumptions when assessing LGB clients.

With every client they have, clinicians should focus on the mental disorder or source of distress not only in the diagnostic stage, but also when assessing treatment progress. Therapists need to be certain that they are assessing progress toward the client's treatment goals (e.g., symptom remission) when assessing progress in therapy, rather than an issue having to do with their sexual orientation. The client's sexual orientation should not enter into the assessment of mental disorders when they initially present at the clinic or during the course of therapy through termination.

Diagnosis

Diagnostics are part of the assessment process, and even though homosexuality has been taken out of the DSM, prejudice may still exist in practice. The possibility of therapist prejudice (e.g., viewing homosexuality as a mental illness) should be considered during the diagnostic process, and appropriate caution should be taken to avoid this view of homosexuality as a mental illness. For example, a homosexual man who has lost his job due to discrimination or experienced a hate crime may experience a lot of distress, which could act as a negative life event to trigger a major depressive episode. Here it is important to attribute the distress to the negative life event rather than to the person's sexual orientation. It is emphasized that scientific tough mindedness and hypothesis testing using objective facts and diagnostic criteria are of the utmost importance. The natural human temptation to reason and attribute to salient features of the person (e.g., the client's sexuality) can only be overridden by systematic examination of the data.

Finally, the therapist's stance towards clients should be LGB-affirming rather than disapproving. Therapists should try to remain objective and focus on what is necessary to reach the goals of diagnosis – typically including acceptance and respect for the client's views of their own sexuality. When Alfred Kinsey described his research on human sexuality, he captured the essence of sound assessment, "We are the recorders and reporters of facts – not the judges of the behaviors we describe."[24]

Treatment

At the beginning of the therapeutic process, building rapport with the client is important for motivation and treatment success. The therapist's knowledge of

LGB issues may be particularly important in building rapport with LGB clients. This may be especially true in light of some psychologists' history of attempting to treat homosexuality as a mental illness.[11] Therapists need to be aware of their own prejudices and be aware of potential harm when building rapport and in the treatment course (e.g., showing disapproval with facial expression or discomfort talking about homosexual activity). Being mindful of one's biases and prejudice is important in the working with LGB clients, because any slight discomfort on the part of the therapist may make the client feel ill at ease or mistrusting of the therapist. For therapists who have negative views of LGB clients, education and consultation with supervisors and peers is recommended. If the clinician still feels that their biases may interfere with responsible and ethical treatment of LGB clients, they are encouraged to refer LGB clients to another service provider who will be able to provide appropriate services for them.

Many currently used empirically supported treatments focus on basic human processes, and therefore should be effective with clients of various backgrounds. They may require little adaptation because the many empirically supported treatments provide a skill set and the framework for change, and at the same time allow flexibility in that the client chooses the content. For example, cognitive-behavioral therapies[25] focus on utilizing empirical information to change maladaptive cognitions. This process of finding evidence for and against maladaptive thoughts can be applied to cognitions on an array of topics. LGB clients may experience cognitions revolving around the special issues that LGB individuals face as a minority group (e.g., their family of origin disapproving of their sexual orientation), but the process by which they can challenge these maladaptive cognitions would remain the same. Similarly, techniques such as behavioral activation[26] and exposure for anxiety disorders[27] should work without adaptation with LGB clients, because of their effects on basic human processes.

Cognitive behavioral therapy (CBT) can be used to challenge maladaptive cognitions about the self through empirical evidence, rather than through a particular value system. For example, one client in our clinic reported he thought, "None of my friends will like me any more if they find out I am gay." CBT could be used to challenge this cognition. The therapist could help the client to identify this as a distortion (e.g., "fortunetelling," "all-or-nothing thinking")[28] and help the client to generate evidence for or against this thought. For instance, perhaps the client's friends have other gay friends, or the client could talk to other LGB people about how their friends reacted when they disclosed that they were gay. Psychologists may also serve as a resource for accurate information about sexual orientation by providing clients with access to empirical data on such topics as the biological data on sexual orientation and statistics about mental health of LGB people and their children.

Other empirically supported therapeutic techniques may be useful in this population. For example, Motivational Interviewing (MI),[29] which is traditionally used for substance use disorders but can be used to enhance desire to change behavior in general, focuses on clarifying what is important to the client and how the client feels, and therefore should be generalizable to LGB clients. In addition, Interpersonal Psychotherapy (IPT),[30] a technique that focuses on interpersonal context of depression, contains a role transitions module that may be useful for an LGB client who has recently decided to disclose that they are homosexual. IPT is well-suited to aid the individual in processing feelings associated with the change in roles and relationships that may result on disclosing his or her sexual orientation. For instance, one client decided to come out to his parents, and mourned the loss of his former role as a heterosexual, married son who matched their longstanding expectations for how he would live his life.

Finally, Cognitive Behavioral Analysis System of Psychotherapy (CBASP)[31] should also generalize to LGB clients, because of the focus on what the client desires as an outcome of a given situation (*see* the comprehensive case illustration for more details on this therapeutic approach). Thus, the content is individualized for each client within a generic framework of each of the aforementioned empirically supported treatments. The presence of the societal stigma associated with homosexuality and bisexuality may also lead to maladaptive cognitions and views of oneself in LGB clients that interfere with them reaching their desired outcomes. CBASP focuses on what the individual wants, so it is guided by the client's values. CBASP can be used as an objective method to help the client to determine what they want from their interpersonal interactions without the therapist's own values being projected.

For example, one of our LGB clients described a situation in which her desired outcome was to tell her sister that she was a lesbian. One of her thoughts was, "I am going to hell because I am gay." CBASP was utilized to identify whether this thought was helpful or hurtful in terms of her chances of reaching her desired outcome. The client identified that this thought was hurtful because it would make it less likely that she would feel enough courage to tell her sister that she was a lesbian. The therapy session then focused on remediation of this hurtful thought. The therapist and client worked together to generate thoughts that would be helpful to her reaching her goal of telling her sister about her sexual orientation (e.g., "My sister loves me very much.").

THE CURRENT STATE OF THE LITERATURE
Assessment

There is some support in the literature for the notion that therapists may mistakenly attribute distress to sexual orientation rather than stress associated with the societal stigma of being an LGB person,[5] and still conceptualize homosexuality and bisexuality as a mental illness that needs to be cured through therapy. For example, Liszcz and Yarhouse[32] conducted a survey among doctoral-level psychologists that involved presenting them with clinical vignettes describing a client who was experiencing same-sex attraction. The psychologists were asked to select the course of action that they viewed as the "best a clinician could make from a professional ethics perspective". Clinicians who were affiliated with a Christian psychology organization were significantly more likely to disagree with a client's desire to "come out of the closet" and significantly more likely to agree with a client's wishes to undergo therapy focused on changing his sexual orientation than psychologists not affiliated with a religious association for psychology and therapists who specialize in LGB issues. This study suggests that LGB individuals who present for therapy may have had negative therapeutic experiences in the past or have had therapists who attributed their problems to their sexual orientation. The study above demonstrates how clinicians may structure treatment goals based on their own beliefs and desires, rather than focusing on clarifying the client's goals and affirming what the client feelings about the situation.

There is some empirical support for the notion that clinicians should not assume that therapy with an LGB client will necessarily include discussion of sexual orientation, and that this focus might actually be harmful to clients. In one of few clinical trials involving a sample of lesbian women, Lewis et al.[33] adapted an expressive writing intervention that had demonstrated effectiveness in reducing distress and improving health in individuals dealing with traumatic events or stressors[34] to target "lesbian-related stressors". The intervention involved a sample of lesbian women writing about traumatic events related to sexual orientation over a two-month period, in the hope that it might be an effective tool for improving health in lesbian women. Interestingly, the intervention successfully reduced self-reports of confusion and stress over the two-month period for lesbian women who were less open about sexual orientation. However, the intervention appeared to have a negative impact on lesbian women who were already open about their sexual orientation prior to the intervention – they had increases in stress and confusion. This study is a salient sample of the potential danger involved with assuming that a situation (in this case, sexual orientation) is going to be traumatic to an individual. Clinicians should be mindful of the power of human resilience through hardship in the majority of cases, and avoid having an iatrogenic effect on LGB individuals.

Diagnosis

A useful way to improve accuracy of diagnosis is for the clinician to consider base rates of a mental disorder in certain populations when making diagnostic judgments.[35] To do this for the treatment of this population, the clinician should be knowledgeable about the rates of mental illness among LGB individuals. Cochran et al.[4] conducted a nationally representative survey (n = 2,917 adults) with the purpose of evaluating potential differences in psychological distress, psychiatric disorders, and use of mental health services among LGB individuals as compared with heterosexual individuals. The homosexual and bisexual women and homosexual and bisexual men were combined for the analysis to increase power, as there were low rates of homosexual and bisexual orientation in the sample. The results indicated that LGB participants had higher rates of psychiatric distress, disorders, and more frequent use of mental health services. However, it is important to emphasize that approximately 60.2% of the LGB group did *not* have any evidence of the five psychiatric disorders assessed (generalized anxiety disorder, major depressive disorder, panic disorder, alcohol dependence, substance dependence) as compared with 83.3% of the heterosexual group. Still, there were higher prevalence rates of mood, anxiety, and substance use disorders when bisexual and homosexual participants were compared with the heterosexual participants of the same gender. The results indicated that gay/bisexual men had higher rates of depression, panic attacks, and psychological distress then heterosexual men. On the other hand, lesbian/bisexual women had higher rates of generalized anxiety disorder than heterosexual women. Moreover, there were higher rates of comorbid disorders among LGB individuals than heterosexual individuals (i.e., LGB people were three to four times more likely to have comorbid psychiatric disorders than heterosexual people of the same gender).[4] Thus, clinicians should consider a greater likelihood of comorbid disorders during the diagnostic process with LGB clients.

In addition to the disorders mentioned above, there is some empirical evidence that homosexual men may be at greater risk than heterosexual men for developing eating disorder symptoms such as drive for thinness and body dissatisfaction.[36-38] One large-scale study found that gay/bisexual adolescent boys were more likely than heterosexual adolescent boys to engage in binge eating and to aspire to look like men in the media.[39] In contrast, some studies suggest that homosexual women may be somewhat buffered from particular disordered eating behaviors such as drive for thinness and use of exercise to control weight.[40] Adolescent girls who identify as bisexual or lesbian also appear to be less prone to body dissatisfaction and less likely to try to look like women in the media than heterosexual girls.[39] Despite lower rates of particular eating disorder symptoms (e.g., drive for thinness), some studies suggest that adult homosexual women do not differ from adult heterosexual women on measures of bulimic symptoms, body dissatisfaction, or weight concerns.[39,41]

Multiple studies suggest that LGB adolescents are at increased risks for suicide attempts compared with heterosexual adolescents.[42,43] Wichstrom and Hegna[43] conducted a large population-based study in Norway with 2,924 participants (grades 7–12) and found that suicide attempts tended to occur at the time the individual realized that they were not exclusively heterosexual. Hypotheses given for this connection were: internalized homophobia, increased risk of bullying, poor social support, and uncertainty/hopelessness about their future. Future studies designed to deepen our understanding of the mechanisms behind the increased rates of suicidal ideation and attempts in LGB adolescents are clearly warranted. In the mean time, the data suggest that clinicians providing services for LGB adolescents may want to carefully assess suicidality, given the heightened risk. This is particularly true if the adolescent has already "come out" or is in the process of "coming out."

Another study compared a group of bisexual and homosexual youth with youngsters from middle and high school on suicidal ideation and suicide attempt status.[42] The study found that homosexual or bisexual orientation doubled the risk for suicidal ideation compared with heterosexual youth, and quadrupled the risk for a suicide attempt compared with heterosexual peers. There was also a main effect for gender, such that being a homosexual or bisexual female particularly increased the risk for suicide attempts. Having peers who were homosexual seemed to reduce the risk for suicidal ideation. The factors highlighted in this study should be considered when conducting risk assessment for suicidal behavior in LGB youth, in addition to using an empirically informed method for categorizing risk.[44]

To reiterate, the fact that there are elevated rates of psychiatric disorders in the LGB population does not imply that being homosexual or bisexual is a mental illness. This is evidenced by two important empirical facts: (i) the majority of LGB individuals do *not* have a psychiatric disorder[4] and (ii) the correlation between mental disorders and sexual orientation is reduced when controlling for stressors that LGB individuals are more likely to encounter, such as discrimination and violence.[17] Therefore, the elevated rates of mental disorders should be conceptualized as a negative consequence of a society that discriminates against a minority group, rather than as a flaw of the individual who is affected by the discrimination.

Treatment

There is a paucity of empirical research on treating LGB clients with specific treatments. Often, clinical trials do not include data on sexual orientation, and researchers do not typically evaluate whether sexual orientation had an impact on treatment outcome. There is no theoretical reason to believe that empirically supported treatments would not work with LGB clients in a similar fashion to heterosexual clients, because the techniques seem to act on fundamental human processes, as mentioned earlier. Clearly, this is an empirical question in need of systematic data.

Despite the improbability of the specific treatment varying in effectiveness based on sexual orientation, it is reasonable to assume that issues that affect motivation to adhere to treatment in all clients, such as rapport, will affect treatment outcome in LGB clients as well. Therapists should pay special attention to perspective-taking with the client and recognize that the client's perspective may have unique aspects that are connected to being an LGB individual. For example, therapists should be aware of special considerations when working with LGB clients (e.g., identity development, being a LGB parent, prejudice) or particular biases that could exist when assessing, diagnosing, and treating LGB clients.[5]

Pachankis and Goldfried[5] suggest that mental health problems may manifest in homosexual and bisexual individuals more often because they have internalized societal homophobia. They suggest that sexual minority individuals may manifest this internalized homophobia through substance misuse, anxiety, and depression symptoms. They propose that LGB individuals who have strong social support through their family and peers, and who are around and have more friends who are also LGB, may be somewhat buffered from developing mental health problems. This hypothesis stresses the importance of the APA's guidelines recommending that therapists are aware of local resources for LGB individuals, so that LGB clients can be referred to them. Social support has been demonstrated as a buffer from mental illness in general, so it stands to reason that it could serve as a protective factor for LGB individuals. Future research should examine the potentially preventive role of social support against mental illness among LGB individuals, because it could have important implications for treatment approaches.

As mentioned above, LGB individuals' experiences with therapy and the therapist can shape their motivation and the effectiveness of treatment. It is suggested that even inadvertent discrimination might negatively impact therapy with LGB individuals. This is supported in analog studies that have found negative effects of subtle discrimination in therapy with LGB clients.[6] In a study looking at LGB individuals' experience of therapy, Liddle[45] found that LGB clients tended to rate heterosexual women and LGB female and male therapists as more helpful to them than heterosexual male therapists, a finding that replicated the results of a previous study.[46] Liddle[45] proposed that this result might be due to the relatively consistent finding that men have more negative attitudes toward LGB people than women.[47]

Because therapists cannot easily change variables such as their gender or sexual orientation, Liddle[45] also examined malleable behaviors that therapists can exhibit. Liddle[45] evaluated 13 suggested guidelines for practice with LGB clients.[6] Nine were inappropriate practices (e.g., "Your therapist gave some indication that s/he assumed you were heterosexual before you indicated your sexual orientation"; "Your therapist blamed your sexual orientation for your problems or insisted on focusing on your sexual orientation without evidence that your sexual orientation was relevant to your problems"; "Your therapist gave you some indication that having a gay or lesbian identity was bad, sick, or inferior"; "Your therapist argued against or pushed you to renounce your sexual identification as a lesbian or gay man"; "Your therapist suddenly refused to see you any more once you disclosed your sexual orientation") and four statements were exemplary practices (e.g., "Your therapist was not afraid to deal with your sexual orientation when it was relevant"; "Your therapist made you feel good about yourself as a gay or lesbian"; "Your therapist was quite knowledgeable about lesbian and gay communities and other resources"). Of the 13 suggested guidelines, 12 were significantly related to overall outcomes of therapy, as indicated by termination of therapy after one session and overall rated helpfulness. The one statement that was not found to be statistically significant in predicting outcome was, "You believed that your therapist did not recognize the importance of lesbian/gay relationships and/or did not appropriately support these relationships."

Liddle's[45] findings suggested that the significantly correlated therapeutic behaviors be addressed in training programs. Furthermore, the findings suggest that there are concrete skills that can make the therapeutic process more culturally sensitive with regard to LGB clients. It could therefore be beneficial for LGB clients that therapists develop these skills. Future research should investigate whether training in these practices enhances therapist effectiveness with LGB clients.

COMPREHENSIVE CASE ILLUSTRATION

Joseph was a 21-year-old college student majoring in music, who was court ordered to an outpatient clinic for therapy as the result of being charged with driving under the influence of alcohol. He was assigned a minimum of 10 sessions of therapy, but this could be extended at the discretion of the therapist if he refused to engage in treatment. He initially presented at the clinic with a guarded interaction style, as evidenced by a defensive validity scale profile on the second edition of the Minnesota Multiphasic Personality Inventory (MMPI-2).[48] Joseph had no scale elevations suggestive of distress or psychological symptomatology (he elevated only Scale 5: Masculinity/Femininity, which, although considered a clinical scale, is not a scale that assesses psychopathology). He also tended to underreport the severity of his drinking habits in therapy compared with the report he gave to a court evaluator. For example, he reported to his therapist that he drank about four beers per week, but he reported to the court evaluator that he drank about eight beers per week. However, with gentle probing about the inconsistencies in his self-report, the inconsistencies were reconciled and the evidence supported a diagnosis of alcohol misuse. He endorsed no anxious or depressive symptomatology or problematic drug use on any of the various symptom measures that were administered at screening: the Beck Anxiety Inventory (BAI),[49] the Beck Depression Inventory-II (BDI),[50] and Short Michigan Alcohol Screening Tool (SMAST).[51] The therapist hypothesized that, because Joseph was a court-ordered client whose progress would be reported to his probation officer, he had a motive to portray himself in an overly positive light. The therapist tested this hypothesis when giving Joseph feedback regarding his MMPI-2 profile and other measures by asking if his response pattern accurately depicted his test-taking attitude and whether or not he had any other ideas as to why a defensive response pattern emerged. Joseph responded that he was indeed hesitant to volunteer any information about his mental health because he was not sure who would see the information (in particular, he worried that his judge or probation officer might see it) and because he did not want anyone to think there was "something wrong with" him just because he had to go to therapy. The therapist's hypothesis that Joseph was withholding information was therefore supported.

Joseph also stated an unwillingness to engage in therapy due to a past negative experience with therapy in which he was counseled for a short time by a psychiatrist whom Joseph found to be self-absorbed and presumptuous about Joseph's feelings and beliefs, and because treatment was mandatory. Therefore, the primary treatment approach used with Joseph was Motivational Interviewing (MI), a therapeutic technique used to elicit motivation for behavior change by exploring the costs and benefits. This treatment approach was utilized to decrease his defensiveness and increase his motivation to engage in therapy. In particular, Joseph and his therapist examined the "problem" of being mandated to attend therapy. They discussed the facts of the situation:

- ▪ weekly therapy sessions were going to cost him a lot of money
- ▪ he had to spend an hour a week in a room with a therapist
- ▪ and his level of cooperation would be evaluated and reported to his probation officer, among others.

His options were delineated:

1. He could not attend therapy.
2. He could attend, but not engage in therapy.
3. He could attend and engage in therapy.

The pros and cons of each option were examined nonjudgmentally. For example, a pro and a con for option 1 were that he would save the money otherwise spent on treatment but he would violate probation. For option 2, he would complete his requirements of probation, but risk an eventual negative evaluation likely resulting in a longer stay in therapy. For option 3, he might learn something in therapy that woulld help him solve issues in his life that he felt were problematic, but he might have to discuss very personal things to accomplish this. At the end of three sessions of MI, Joseph decided that, as long as he had to be in therapy and was spending his own money on it, he may as well engage and see what he could get out of it.

Next, it was established that treatment would have to include discussion of Joseph's drinking habits and what factors contribute to his problematic drinking. The rationale for this treatment decision was that he was court ordered to therapy for the purpose of addressing his problematic drinking, and the reports that the therapist would send to his probation officer had to report that this issue was being addressed or he would not meet his probation requirements. However, to maintain his motivation to engage in therapy, Joseph and his therapist agreed that his therapy sessions could include a productive discussion on any issue in his life he wanted to "work on". After some discussion of potential topics, Joseph shared that he was attracted to men and women and engaged in sexual behavior with people of both sexes. Further, he stated that he would like to spend the time in therapy working on this aspect of his life. When asked to elaborate (i.e., to describe what about his attraction to men and women he wanted to "work on"), he stated that he was concerned with the potential negative reaction of his heterosexual friends if he told them he was attracted to men. In addition, regarding those friends who were aware of his bisexual orientation, he stated that he experienced a lot of pressure from his gay male friends to "be gay", and from his heterosexual friends to "be straight". Last, he described himself as effeminate and experienced pressure to "tone it down" when he was around friends to whom he was not out.

Before continuing the case study, two points regarding scientific mindedness and dynamic sizing are worthy of highlighting. First, it must be noted that this therapist, although likely aware of common stereotypes about gay men, exerted restraint in applying these stereotypes to his client. For example, the therapist made no assumptions about his sexual orientation based on the fact that his client was a fine arts major and that he endorsed little concern in traditionally masculine interests, as evidenced by an elevated 5 MMPI-2 code type. Had the therapist allowed himself to be influenced by his knowledge of stereotypes about gay men, he may have also assumed that Joseph's defensiveness was due to a fear of negative judgments by the therapist due to his sexual orientation and explored this hypothesis (without reason to do so). Had this occurred, the therapist may have unwittingly alienated an already disengaged client early on in the therapy process. Second, after Joseph shared his sexual orientation with his therapist, the therapist did not assume that Joseph meant that his sexual orientation *per se* was the problem he wanted to address. Rather, the therapist asked Joseph to elaborate on his statement, and learned that Joseph wanted to "work on" the anxiety he was experiencing during his coming out process as a result of the pressure from his friends that he experienced and feared. In other words, the therapist learned that it was the societal reaction to his sexual orientation that caused him distress and not his sexual orientation.

After MI had been successfully used to enhance Joseph's motivation for treatment, the primary treatment approach was changed to CBASP to help Joseph identify situational triggers for his problematic drinking, as well as identify those aspects of a situation that made him most fearful of a negative reaction from his peers. In addition, CBASP would be helpful for Joseph to identify more helpful ways of interacting with others that would decrease his vulnerability to problematic drinking and minimize his distress.

Joseph completed weekly homework assignments (Coping Survey Questionnaires [CSQs], which ask for detailed descriptions of his thoughts and behaviors during a brief interpersonal interaction) and in-session exercises that taught him how to conceptualize situations in a CSQ format, such that Joseph could identify his desired outcome, and determine which thoughts and behaviors would increase his chances of achieving his goal for the situation. Throughout therapy, Joseph's situational analyses often involved thoughts about not wanting to appear disloyal to friends or otherwise upset or disappoint his friends. Joseph often stated that his friends were important to him and he did not want them to be upset with him, so if they wanted to him to do something, he usually would do it against his better judgment. This behavior would lead to problematic outcomes such as drinking too much to be able to practice violin the next day, or being pressured to engage in sexual behavior with which he was not comfortable. Later, he would be disappointed with himself for having done these things, leading him to feel like an inadequate violinist and confused about his sexuality. He decided that he wanted to learn how to say no to his friends and others without feeling disloyal. Below is a transcript of a session that discussed the issue.

Therapist (T): So what is your CSQ about this week?

Joseph (J): Well, I went home for the weekend and I went out with an old friend from high school while I was there. I wrote about that.

T: OK. Sounds great. I know your friends are really important to you. Let's start with step 1, describe the situation in a brief, clear way.

J: Ok. During the time Mindy and I were hanging out, we made out and she asked to have sex with me.

T: OK. That's pretty concise and clear now. Let's try step 2. While you and Mindy were making out and she asked to have sex with you, what thoughts were running through your head?

J: Well, she and I had had sex when we were in high school, and she brought up the possibility of having sex now, so I figured I would have sex with Mindy again. Also, I was afraid I'd hurt her feelings if I didn't. Also, because she brought it up, I really wanted her to have a good time.

T: OK. Let me make sure that I have a clear understanding of what was going through your head. I think I heard you describe these three thoughts: (i) I'm going to have sex with Mindy again, (ii) I don't want to hurt her feelings by saying no, and (iii) I want Mindy to enjoy sex with me. Did I understand correctly?

J: Yeah, that's right.

T: OK, so step 3. What were your behaviors in this situation; or rather, what did you do?

J: Well, basically I tried to get an erection but couldn't. I got really nervous and that made things worse.

T: What about step 4: How did the event come out for you – how did it end?

J: Well in the end we didn't have sex and I felt really bad about it. Like I hurt her feelings or something.

T: How did you want the event to come out?

J: I wanted to have and enjoy sex with Mindy.

T: Did you get what you wanted?

J: No!

T: Why not?

J: Because I couldn't get an erection!

T: Alright let's suppose that in spite of getting nervous, being worried that she wouldn't enjoy sex with you, you were still able to get an erection and have sex with Mindy. Would you have gotten what you wanted, which was "to have *and* enjoy sex with Mindy"?

J: Well, I don't know. We would have had sex so "yes" on that part. I don't enjoy doing anything when I feel a lot of pressure to do it or someone might not like it. Like when I'm being tested on the violin.

T: Hmm. That's an interesting thought. Why don't we go back to your thoughts and see how those influenced the outcome too. Let's focus on the part of the outcome about enjoying sex with Mindy now, and let's start with "I'm going to have sex with Mindy." Was thinking that helpful or hurtful to getting you what you wanted, and why?

J: Well, actually it was hurtful, because I felt like I didn't have a choice. It was just going to happen.

T: Hmm. That makes a lot of sense. It's not fun to feel like you don't have a say in what you're doing. What would have been a more helpful thought?

J: How about "I want to have sex with Mindy"?

T: Would that have been helpful for getting you what you wanted, which was to enjoy sex with Mindy?

J: No.

T: Why?

J: Because I didn't want to have sex with Mindy. She wanted to have sex with me.

Remediation of Joseph's other two thoughts went similarly. No interpretation of the situation would lead him to have enjoyed sex with Mindy, because he was only agreeing to have sex because she wanted to. He feared that saying no would hurt her feelings.

T: You know, we gave it a really good go at trying to get you what you wanted, but nothing seemed to work. Why do you suppose that is?

J: I don't know. I guess it would have been hard to enjoy sex with her, if I was just doing it because she wanted to. I have to want it too, and I have to be attracted to her. I just wasn't attracted to Mindy, even though she's a great girl.

T: I'm sure she is. What does that say about the CSQ?

J: I think I was trying to make myself want something I didn't just to avoid making her feel bad.

T: Hmm, like maybe your desired outcome was unattainable?

J: Yeah. There was no way I was going to enjoy sex with her if I was doing it for all the wrong reasons.

T: Hmm, that makes a lot of sense. So what can you take away from your work today?

J: I think I don't have to have sex if I don't want to, and that I probably wouldn't enjoy it anyway if I did it for other reasons. And a good clue that I don't want to is that I'm just not attracted to that person.

T: Hmm, so it's not about who that person is or what other people want? It's about whether or not you want it too and are attracted to that person?

J: Yes. Exactly.

Over time, Joseph learned that his fears of disappointing others led to other problems. He rarely enjoyed playing the violin because he feared his audience would be disappointed by his performance, he would never say no to a drink offered to him by a friend, etc. Therapy also involved having Joseph test his fear of appearing disloyal to friends by doing things like expressing a dissenting opinion, or turning down an invitation to go out, and watching for their reaction. When he would worry about whether or not his behavior appeared disloyal to someone, he would approach the person and ask if they felt he had been disloyal. Most of these exposure exercises led him to believe that many of his worries were unfounded. At the end of 10 sessions of therapy, Joseph had made much progress at identifying situational triggers for drinking and coming up with ways to avoid them. He had completed his court-mandated therapy in the required number of sessions. After that, Joseph decided to continue therapy as a non-court-ordered client and attended another 10 sessions of therapy at our clinic. He was very consistent about completing homework assignments, and began to generate his own homework assignments and therapy goals. At the end of 20 sessions of treatment, Joseph reported an increase in self-esteem and self-efficacy. In addition, his therapist noticed an increase in assertiveness, as he was more willing to correct his therapist whenever the therapist misunderstood him, and was more interested in debating issues with his therapist, rather than asking the therapist what he thought Joseph should do in a given situation.

CONCLUSIONS AND FUTURE DIRECTIONS

The field would greatly benefit from more empirical data on the experience that LGB clients have with psychological services. For example, how often do LGB individuals experience prejudice in assessment, diagnostics, and/or therapy, and what issues are most important for their therapist to know about? In addition to empirical studies focused on evaluating LGB clients' experience in assessment, diagnosis, and therapy, rigorous clinical trials that evaluate the effectiveness of empirically supported treatments (such as CBASP and CBT) in LGB samples would greatly contribute to our understanding of the best services to provide to LGB clients. These data would provide important information, empirically, about whether the same treatments should be used for heterosexual and LGB clients. In addition to evaluating the use of these treatments on mental disorders (e.g., anxiety, depression) in LGB clients, it would be useful to see how helpful these frameworks are with LGB clients who wish to sort through issues of sexual identity.

Safren[52] calls for the integration of empirically supported treatments in combination with the therapist having an affirmative (i.e., positive, approving) stance toward client homosexuality/bisexuality. He stated that many gay-affirmative programs do not utilize empirically supported treatments and vice versa. In the future, programs that involve both empirically supported treatments and an affirmative stance toward homosexuality would probably provide the best services to LGB clients. This chapter has discussed the lack of clear-cut evidence supporting the effectiveness of sexual reorientation therapy. However, as Spitzer[10] points out, there is also no empirical evidence for LGB-affirmative therapy. Empirical studies should be conducted on the usefulness and effectiveness of LGB-affirmative therapy to determine if it is beneficial and/or has any harmful effects. Then, clinicians can feel more certain that they are practicing ethical therapeutic techniques with LGB clients.

In addition to more empirical study in this area, a psychoeducational component on LGB individuals' unique life experiences as part of training programs and continuing education should help therapists to feel and act in a more competent way in serving the needs of this minority group. Pachankis and Goldfried[5] suggest that education on LGB issues be an essential component to clinical training. Without education on LGB issues, therapists are less likely to be competent in working with this population. In the absence of objective information regarding the perspectives of LGB individuals, clinicians may be left to rely on their own biases and personal experiences rather than on science.

Sherry et al.[53] recently contacted 135 clinical programs and 69 counseling programs and requested that they fill out a survey about their program's training on LGB issues. Of the programs that responded, 67.6% required a multicultural course, and 71% of the programs that required a multicultural course included a section on LGB issues. Regarding clinical practicum options, 89.5% of the programs reported providing opportunities for students to do clinical work with LGB clients, and 94.3% of the programs reported covering issues of sexual orientation in clinical supervision. These percentages must be interpreted with some caution, because there was a 51% response rate, and thus a selection bias may have affected the results. The results of this survey suggest that there is a multicultural component to many mental health graduate programs, and it is hoped that 100% of programs will include multicultural competence components in the future. Therapists who are not educated on LGB issues are encouraged to seek supervision and consult with colleagues so that they can provide a proper standard of care to LGB clients.

CHAPTER 5

The Assessment, Diagnosis, and Treatment of Psychiatric Disorders in Religiously Diverse Clients

Jessica S Brown, and Kimberly A Van Orden

For many people seeking treatment, religion is an important and permanent component of life. For others, a change in feelings about faith may be the driving force in seeking treatment. Still other clients may not possess strong religious beliefs that impact their daily life. As clinicians, each of us may have our own beliefs and values with regard to religion. It is important as clinicians that we allow our clients to express their religious beliefs and incorporate them into the therapeutic milieu to the degree they wish.

This chapter will address how religion plays a role in the assessment, diagnosis, and treatment of mental illness. We will discuss issues of both religion and spirituality. Research in this area has not provided a single definition of either of these concepts; rather definitions vary from study to study.[1] Hill and colleagues[2] attempt to conceptually integrate the concepts of religion and spirituality, and suggest that the two concepts are by no means incompatible. In support of this approach are findings that individuals' self-descriptions tend to include labels of both "religious" and "spiritual".[1] Thus many individuals who think of themselves as "religious" also think of themselves as "spiritual" (and vice versa). However, many researchers (and many of the studies described in this chapter) explicitly distinguish between the constructs of religion and spirituality, and many authors recommend making this distinction.[3] Definitions of spirituality often define the spiritual domain as the aspects of life involving transcendental or existential concerns (e.g., reference 4), the search for meaning, purpose, truth, and values (e.g., reference 3), and containing either secular or religious content (e.g., reference 5). Spirituality may be found in diverse domains – through religion; a relationship with a divine being, nature, music, and the arts; a set of values or principles; or a pursuit of scientific knowledge.[3] Although not holding in all circumstances, religious expressions tend to be public, whereas spiritual expressions tend to be private.[4] In this manner, spirituality is often defined as an attribute of individuals, while religion (and religiosity) is defined as the beliefs, rituals, and practices of an institution.[6] As religion may be one avenue for spiritual expression, Richards and Bergin[4] conceptualize religion as a subset of spirituality. In this chapter, we use Richards and Bergin's[4] conceptualization of religion and spirituality as related concepts. For convenience, we use the term "religion" to refer to both spiritual expressions and religious practices (unless noted otherwise).

Should spiritual and religious issues be assessed by mental health professionals? Psychotherapy clients in the United States are likely to be involved in religious organizations. However, the wide variety of religious groups in the United States means that a diverse range of beliefs and practices will be brought to therapy.[7] D'Souza[8] provides data that clients believe that spirituality and religious issues do have a place in mental health treatment: in a survey of Australian psychiatric patients, 82% reported that their therapists should be aware of their spiritual beliefs and needs. A national survey of American adults with mental illness found that 50% of respondents reported that they engaged in religious or spiritual activities that they believed were beneficial to their mental health, such as prayer, attending worship services, and religious/spiritual reading.[9] Client perception that religion/spirituality was a source of motivation for change in drug misuse treatment programs was one dimension that discriminated between groups of recovered versus nonrecovered outpatient methadone treatment clients.[10] Despite indications that clients may desire to discuss religious/spiritual concerns in therapy, Lindgren and Coursey[11] present data that these discussions may not frequently occur: they found that only half of the clients in their sample who reported a desire to discuss religious and spiritual beliefs in therapy also reported perceptions that they were free to do so.

Current data suggest that a large proportion of clients in the United States believe that their therapists should be aware of religious and spiritual concerns (e.g., reference 8), and believe that religious/spiritual activities are beneficial to their mental health (e.g., reference 9). Yet, these issues may not be raised in therapy due to clients' perceptions that the discussions are unwelcome (*cf.* data presented by Lindgren and Coursey[11]) or due to religious clients' distrust in mental health professionals or the process of psychotherapy.[12] Thus, beliefs and behaviors of both the therapist and the client may make it less likely that religion will be discussed in therapy or used in treatment planning. Consideration of religion is a necessary component of culturally sensitive treatments, as it is ultimately an exercise in dynamic sizing, yet religion is not often considered in the assessment, diagnosis, and treatment of mental illness. Thus, one goal of this chapter is to provide a model for incorporating religion into assessment, diagnosis, and treatment in a culturally sensitive manner. To accomplish this, we first discuss how religion may be relevant for assessment, diagnosis, and treatment using case examples from our own community clinic. Next, we provide a brief review of the scientific literature on the role of religion in mental health services. We then discuss a comprehensive case example that brings together the main points in each of the earlier sections.

Finally, we conclude with suggestions for future directions for research and clinical practice.

CLINICAL OBSERVATIONS
Assessment

During the intake assessment, it is important to allow clients to discuss their religious beliefs, and how these beliefs may or may not be relevant to the therapeutic experience. It may be useful to simply ask about religion during the interview, saying something such as "Tell me about your religious beliefs" or "Tell me how spirituality relates to your life". For some people, religion may be a sensitive subject and being asked openly and nonjudgmentally about it by their therapist may make them feel much more comfortable in discussing it.

Discussing religion with a client may also help to build rapport and help the clinician to see the client as a whole person, rather than just someone with a psychological disorder. For some individuals, religion plays a significant role in their life and will come up frequently throughout the therapeutic process. By introducing this issue during the assessment phase, the client can lay the groundwork for discussing religion in future sessions. It also gives the clinician an opportunity to indicate how much he or she knows about the client's religion, and to demonstrate an openness to learning about the client's beliefs. The following case example helps to illustrate this point.

> *Therapist* (*T*): Mark, please tell me how spirituality relates to your life.
>
> *Mark*: Well, I consider myself to be a very religious person. I am Jewish . . . Do you know much about Judaism?
>
> *T*: No, not very much. But I would like to learn more. Could you tell me about the role of Judaism in your life?

The client then goes on to tell the therapist a bit more about his feelings regarding his faith. They also come to an understanding that the clinician should feel free to ask questions about anything the client brings up that is unclear. As the therapy progresses, the client at times will even explain some of the religious practices that he talks about even before the clinician can ask. In this manner, the clinician is able to get a fuller picture of who the client is as an individual and how religion fits into his life. Additionally, religiosity may influence scores on assessment measures such as the Minnesota Multiphasic Personality Inventory-2 (MMPI-2). Research on this topic is discussed later in this chapter.

Diagnosis

Perhaps the most important point to make regarding religious sensitivity in diagnosis is that one should not diagnose as abnormal something that is considered a part of the client's religious practice and does not cause that individual functional impairment. A thorough assessment of the client's religion and typical religious practices will help to make this distinction. In addition, further research into the client's religion may be necessary to confirm what practices are considered normal within that religion, a process akin to Sue's[13] principles of scientific mindedness and dynamic sizing. This will help clinicians make the distinction between whether or not behaviors and beliefs are symptoms of clinical disorders or normal religious practices. This point is so important that the *Diagnostic and Statistical Manual of Mental Disorders*, fourth edition, text revision (DSM-IV-TR) makes a statement regarding the issue:[14] (p. xxxiv)

> "A clinician who is unfamiliar with the nuances of an individual's cultural frame of reference may incorrectly judge as psychopathology those normal variations in behavior, belief, or experience that are particular to the individual's culture. For example, certain religious practices or beliefs (e.g. hearing or seeing a deceased relative during bereavement) may be misdiagnosed as manifestation of a Psychotic Disorder."

Once a clinician has identified potential symptoms, another means of resolving the issue of whether they are normal religious practice or mental illness is to ask the client how distressing and impairing these behaviors or beliefs are. As is noted throughout DSM-IV, full criteria for a disorder are not met unless the client is experiencing clinically significant distress or impairment.[14] If the symptoms being experienced by the client are not distressing or impairing, it is likely that a diagnosis is not warranted. However, it is important to keep in mind that behaviors or beliefs that *are* part of normal religious experience for a client may still cause that client some distress or impairment. For example, consider the case of the individual who hears or sees a deceased relative during bereavement. Although this experience may be normative according to his or her religious practices, it may also cause extreme sadness and grief (i.e., distress) regarding the lost loved one. Therefore, just because a potential symptom causes distress or impairment does not mean that it is not a normative religious experience.

Another situation that may arise during the diagnostic phase is nonacceptance of the diagnosis on the part of the client or the client's family due to religious beliefs. Some religions, such as Roman Catholicism, believe that spirits or the devil may be the cause of abnormal behavior. Therefore, members of these religious groups may be reluctant to accept that a mental illness is the cause of problematic behaviors and thoughts. A young man named Sam with very religious parents presented at our community-based clinic. Given symptoms such as tactile hallucinations, delusions of reference, and inappropriate affect, Sam was diagnosed as having schizophrenia. He had also experienced several suicide attempts and inpatient hospitalizations, but Sam's parents were still reluctant to accept the diagnosis of schizophrenia. His delusions and hallucinations had no religious content or meaning to them, and his parents believed that these thoughts and behaviors were abnormal. However, they did not believe that he was suffering from a mental illness; rather that he had been possessed by the devil and if they prayed enough, he would recover. It was very difficult for the parents to accept that their son was suffering from a severe mental illness and that he needed extensive care. Although it is understandable, perhaps even normative, for parents to have difficulty accepting that their child has a severe mental illness, this family's religious beliefs presented an extra barrier preventing them from coming to terms with their son's diagnosis.

Treatment

First and foremost, treatment should not interfere with faith whenever possible. This statement does not mean that treatment should ignore faith, rather, that the treatment provided should not conflict with the client's faith. A number of therapies meet this requirement. For example, the Cognitive Behavioral Analysis System of Psychotherapy[15] (CBASP) is designed to help clients by having them evaluate situations that occur in their daily lives and determine how to be more successful at achieving their desired outcome in each situation. The client generates his or her own desired outcome for each situation, making this therapy compatible with any religious viewpoint. By allowing the client to set his or her own goals for how situations should be resolved, this treatment ensures that the goals the client is working toward will be compatible with his or her own religious beliefs. In this manner, CBASP is value-free, as the therapist does not make any judgments regarding what outcomes or goals the client works toward.

Another example of a treatment that may effectively work without interfering with religious beliefs is exposure-based treatment for anxiety disorders. In this type of treatment, the therapist and client work together to generate a list of feared situations that the client would like to be able to experience without impairing or distressing levels of anxiety. The client is able to set the parameters of the situations and the therapist does not force the client to complete any specific exposures that he or she is unwilling to complete. Take, for example, a client diagnosed with obsessive compulsive disorder (OCD) who spends 8–10 hours each day praying. Although praying is an important part of this individual's religion, it is also interfering with her ability to be successful in life – to hold down a job and to have friendships and romantic relationships. This client expressed to her therapist that she would like to be able to pray less frequently, yet still pray daily. The client and therapist worked together using the techniques of exposure with response prevention[16] to gradually decrease the amount of time spent in prayer each day and increase the time spent in social activities.

Alternatively, a therapist may have a client diagnosed with OCD who is more concerned with other rituals such as cleaning or checking and not distressed about the time that they spend praying. With this client, exposure treatment could focus on the other rituals and not target the prayer rituals, again illustrating the role of dynamic sizing. If the client is not distressed or impaired by their prayer rituals, there is no therapeutic reason to try to change them. Just like CBASP, exposure treatments may have heightened success with people from diverse religious backgrounds, as they allow the clients to set their own goals and work toward them in a way that is compatible with their religious beliefs. They also ensure that the clinician does not have to place a value judgment on the client's actions.

Although it is important that treatment does not conflict with faith, at times treatment may be focused on issues of faith. Clients may seek treatment to help deal with conflicts of faith, such as personal disagreement with general church doctrines or questions about their own faith-based belief systems. In those cases, therapy can be helpful as an opportunity for the client to discuss these issues freely and work out a way to reconcile personal values with religious values. For these clients, it is important to provide a supportive, nonjudgmental environment to allow them to explore their own feelings. Therapies such as Interpersonal Psychotherapy[17] (IPT) may be useful in these circumstances. IPT has four areas of focus, one of which is role transition. For a client who has been a strong believer in a specific organized religion but is shifting to creating his or her own system of spirituality and values, IPT role transition is a useful tool to help facilitate that transition. However, it is also important for a therapist to not force a focus on faith when the client is presenting in treatment primarily to seek help with other issues. The therapist must be careful to allow clients to discuss spirituality when desired but not bring it up repeatedly if the client does not identify it as a focal point of therapy.

Finally, the therapist's own religious viewpoints should be taken into consideration during treatment. It is important for the therapist to not force his or her own views onto the client and to not make pronouncements about the client's behavior based on the perspective of the therapist's religion. Clients, particularly those who are very spiritual themselves, may ask about a therapist's own religious background or knowledge of a specific religion. The therapist should address these issues openly and honestly, but not discuss them at length, as the client's situation is the primary focus of therapy. Lengthy discussion of the therapist's religious views may serve to make the client feel that he or she will be judged by the therapist. Consider the case of a lesbian woman who seeks therapy to work through problems with her long-time partner. If she asks her therapist about his religion and he talks at length about how he is a strict Catholic, she may feel much less comfortable discussing her sexual orientation with him. Once again, therapists must focus on working toward the client's goals rather than the goals that they think may be appropriate for their client. The following case example illustrates how a therapist may wish to respond to questions regarding his or her own religious views.

Sarah (S): So, Tom, what religion do you adhere to?

Therapist (T): Sarah, I'm willing to talk with you about my spirituality if you really want to know about it, but I think that it is important for us to remember that I'm here to help you to explore the issues that you are interested in overcoming.

S: Well, I was just wondering.

T: Why were you wondering?

S: In the past I've found that people of certain religious groups tended to be judgmental about things. So I guess I'm wondering about how you might judge me.

T: I see. That's certainly a valid concern. But let me assure you that I feel my role as your therapist is to help you reach whatever goals you have, and my own personal feelings or value judgments are irrelevant to that process. Is there something in particular that is bothering you that people have been judgmental about in the past?

In this example, the therapist was able to explain to Sarah that his chief concern as her therapist was to help her to improve herself and that he intended to be nonjudgmental. He was also able to get Sarah talking about something else that was bothering her, namely, the issue of being judged by others. Whereas sometimes clients ask personal questions of their therapists out of mere curiosity, at other times the client has a larger issue in mind. Finding out why the client is asking the question may open up an important avenue of discussion.

THE CURRENT STATE OF THE LITERATURE

As mentioned above, spirituality is an important dimension of culturally sensitive therapies.[18] The following section briefly reviews the literature on religion and mental health. Our goal is to answer (at least in part) what is involved in culturally sensitive treatment with regard to diversity in religion and spirituality. This review is by no means exhaustive: a selective emphasis is placed on empirical contributions to the literature. In addition, although we do not mean to suggest that treatment considerations are necessarily the same for those of all religious and spiritual beliefs and practices, the present review does not attempt to comprehensively address specific treatment considerations for particular religions. Instead we use selective examples to illustrate general principles. Readers interested in treatment considerations and recommendations for specific religious affiliations may wish to consult Koenig[19] as well as Richards and Bergin.[20] The latter text dedicates individual chapters to the major religions represented in America, including breakdowns by denominations, (e.g., there are separate chapters for Roman Catholicism and Eastern Orthodox Christianity). Each chapter begins with an overview of the beliefs and practices of the religion for readers who desire general information about religious groups in addition to specific treatment guidelines, as a way to help build up culture-specific expertise.

Assessment

The finding presented above that clients often do not discuss religion with therapists despite a desire to do so suggests that methods of assessing religious/spiritual issues and concerns need to facilitate client acceptability and trust as well as provide information that will aid in treatment. A common recommendation in the literature is for therapists to take a *spiritual history* (e.g., references 21 and 22) or *spiritual assessment* (e.g., reference 3) with clients during the intake or assessment phase of treatment. General areas to assess include clients' levels of identification and involvement with the religious or spiritual tradition. Another goal of spiritual assessment or spiritual history is to assess whether religious/spiritual practices are normative (relative to others who share the same beliefs and practices) and whether they are used in a healthy or unhealthy manner.[12] In some cases, the influence of religious/spiritual beliefs and practices may be apparent during the development of psychopathology (e.g., symptoms with religious content), whereas in others the influence of religious/spiritual beliefs may be apparent during the prevention or treatment of psychopathology. An assessment of religious/spiritual beliefs and practices is thus part of a thorough assessment which may aid in a therapist's understanding of the client's problems as well as the identification of potential client resources that may facilitate treatment.[22]

Koenig and Weaver[23] provide a general framework to use in a spiritual history that is based on a list of psychological and spiritual needs of clients, each of which may be addressed. The framework includes three categories, "needs related to self" (e.g., a need for meaning and purpose), "needs related to God" (e.g., a need to experience the presence of God), and "needs related to others" (e.g., a need for fellowship with others). Baez and Hernandez[24] suggest that assessments of spiritual belief systems need to be dynamic and include a range of beliefs and practices. Including the assessment of a range of spiritual beliefs would prevent simplistic categorizations of individuals into "believes" or "does not believe" groups.

More specific recommendations and assessment tools are available to guide therapists in taking a spiritual history. For example, Puchalski and Romer[21] suggest completing four steps when completing a spiritual history. The steps can be remembered with the acronym, "FICA." The first step ("F" for *faith*) involves asking questions related to the client's faith and beliefs, such as whether they consider themselves spiritual or religious and if they have spiritual beliefs that aid in coping with stress. The second step ("I" for *importance*) involves questions related to the importance of faith and beliefs in the client's life, such as what role beliefs play in the client's actions toward recovery. The third step ("C" for *communities*) involves questions about the clients' involvement in spiritual or religious communities. The final step ("A" for *address*) involves questions about how clients would like their therapist to address the issues they described in treatment. Anandarajah and Hight[3] provide a similar set of questions for a spiritual assessment, denoted by the acronym "HOPE." The first set of questions ("H" for *hope*) addresses sources of hope, comfort, and strength for clients. The second set ("O" for *organized*) address clients' level of participation in organized religion. The third set ("P" for *personal practices*) addresses personal spiritual practices. The fourth set ("E" for *effects*) addresses the effects of spirituality on treatment. We are not aware of research demonstrating that the use of these spiritual assessment tools directly improves accuracy of diagnosis or treatment outcomes. Our recommendation on the use of these assessment tools therefore remains tentative, though it appears that the use of these tools may help clinicians to implement dynamic sizing more appropriately.

Over 100 standardized measures of religiousness and spirituality are available. A review of all of these measures is not possible here; interested readers are referred to Hill and Hood,[25] and Slater et al.,[26] both of which provide information on measures of religiousness and spirituality. Some of these measures assess parts of the religiousness or spirituality (as opposed to the global frameworks discussed above, such as "FICA" and "HOPE"). For example, the Spiritual Transcendence Scale[27] (STS) assesses the capacity of individuals to engage in "spiritual transcendence" – a behavior that involves three parts – universality, connectedness, and prayer fulfillment. the STS has been shown to predict such psychological variables as wellbeing, stress experience, and psychological growth.[6] These variables may be relevant to treatment outcome. For example, diagnoses or symptom counts are often used as outcomes in studies of psychological treatments; however, an individual's wellbeing at the end of treatment may also represent a relevant outcome variable (e.g., see reference 28). In addition, an individual's response to psychotherapy might depend on his or her experiences of stress or levels of psychological growth, both of which may be influenced by religion and spirituality.

There is also evidence that religion and spirituality may impact clients' responses to standard assessment measures (i.e., those designed to measure mental health symptoms, not religion or spirituality). For example, one study found religious participation and spirituality were associated with responses on the MMPI-2.[29] These researchers found that individuals who reported religious involvement obtained lower clinical scale scores than individuals who reported no religious involvement. These results indicate that religious individuals responded to the questions on the MMPI-2 in a way that suggests lower levels of psychopathology. These data suggest that clinicians may need to consider religion and spirituality when interpreting standard assessment measures.

Diagnosis

Many researchers suggest that religiosity/spirituality should be considered when diagnosing psychopathology in clients: beliefs and practices may be used in either adaptive or maladaptive ways (e.g., references 12, 30, and 31). Therefore, therapists must determine whether maladaptive religious/spiritual beliefs and practices may be contributing to the development or maintenance of a disorder (e.g., reference 32) or may be influencing the content of symptoms (e.g., reference 33). Sahlein[30] suggests that therapists use their scientific mindedness and begin by hypothesizing about whether religious/spiritual beliefs and practices are promoting or impeding mental health.

Research supports the hypothesis that religious/spiritual beliefs and practices may influence the content and expression of a disorder, rather than directly contributing to the development or maintenance of a disorder. For example, level of religiosity was not predictive of the presence of religious obsessions in a sample of individuals with OCD. This finding suggests that higher levels of religiosity did not lead to the development of symptoms.[34] However, in the same sample, in individuals who did present with a variety of obsessions, religious obsessions were common. The authors suggest that religion is one domain in which OCD manifests itself rather than religion being a cause of the disorder. Greenberg and Witztum[31] suggest two domains in which religion may contribute to the content of OCD symptoms – cleanliness and purity, and liturgy. The religious theme of cleanliness and purity may appear in the content of obsessions such as dirt and contamination, or compulsive behaviors such as washing. Religious liturgy, especially prayer and confession, may also appear in the content of obsessions and compulsions (e.g., guilt association with confession among Roman Catholic individuals with OCD). Religious content also appears in the content of bipolar I symptoms; for example, Jerrell and Shugart[35] found that hyper-religiosity was found in 18.5% of a sample of adults with bipolar I disorder. Finally, Wilson[33] suggests that religion may "color the expression of symptoms" in both schizophrenia and affective disorders, but that religion is unlikely to serve as a causal mechanism in the development of a disorder (p. 172).

The literature reviewed above suggests that religious content may appear in the symptoms of disorders such as OCD, bipolar I disorder, and schizophrenia. When are religious practices better described as expressions of faith and belief and when are they better described as symptoms of a disorder? Greenberg and Witztum[31] suggest that religious content which is repetitive in nature and handled pedantically is most likely to appear as a focus of symptoms. Based on their observations (not empirical data), they suggest that the practice of religious rituals is likely to be symptomatic of a disorder when the following conditions are present: the behavior exceeds the requirements of religious law, the behavior is concentrated solely on one particular area (not an overall concern for religious practice), a narrow focus leads to neglect of other features of religious life, or rituals are repeated solely due to fear that a ritual was omitted.

Religion or spirituality has also been found to relate to the number and severity of mental health symptoms with which a client presents. For example, Murphy and colleagues[36] found that stronger religious beliefs predicted lower levels of depressive symptoms in clients with clinical depression; this effect was due to lower levels of hopelessness among religious individuals. Thus, religious individuals reported less depression and this relationship was explained by the fact that religious individuals were less hopeless. The authors suggest that one interpretation of their findings is that the presence of religious beliefs may counteract negative thoughts that lead to hopelessness and depression. However, this study used a cross-sectional design; thus, we cannot conclude that religiosity caused less hopelessness or less depression. In a similar study, Baetz and colleagues[37] investigated the relation of frequency of worship attendance to mental health outcomes in a sample of psychiatric inpatients. More frequent worship attendance was related to less severe depressive symptoms, shorter hospitalization stays, higher satisfaction with life, and lower current and lifetime alcohol misuse. In addition, involvement in a religious community was found to be associated with lowered rates of antisocial behavior (i.e., lifetime violence, delinquency, and status offenses) in a sample of adolescents.[38] Thus, the likelihood of obtaining a diagnosis may depend on a client's level of religious or spiritual involvement.

Why might religious and spiritual variables relate to mental health outcomes? One process suggested in the literature is religious coping – the use of religious beliefs and practices to provide comfort, hope, and meaning in times of distress.[39] In a cross-sectional examination of religious coping in a sample of psychiatric inpatients, increased time spent on religious coping (e.g., prayer or reading the Bible) was related to lower levels of frustration and less severe symptomatology.[40] Identification of processes such as religious coping provides a potential explanation for the relation between religion/spirituality and mental health outcomes.

A final area relevant to formulating a diagnosis involves the issues or concerns about religion or spirituality that clients bring to therapy as a potential focus of therapy. The DSM-IV-TR includes codes for conditions or problems that may be a focus of clinical attention but that are not considered disorders; these conditions and problems are coded on axis I. The DSM-IV-TR provides a specific code for religious or spiritual problems (V62.89). Examples of concerns that may fall under this category include distress concerning loss or questioning of faith, problems associated with the conversion to a new faith, or questioning of spiritual values that may not be related to a religious institution.

Treatment

A large number of studies on the relation between religion and physical health conducted with diverse samples, differing designs and methods, different measures, and diverse types of health outcomes, converge on the finding that religious involvement and affiliation are associated with positive physical outcomes, including lowered risk for cardiovascular disease, hypertension, and stroke.[41,42] Studies generally also find a positive relation between religion and mental health outcomes.[42] One review of the relation between religion and mental health outcomes with over 200 studies found a positive relation between religion and mental health outcomes in approximately half of the studies and a negative association in fewer than a quarter of the studies.[43] The data thus far indicate that religion and spirituality are related to mental health outcomes. Religion and spirituality most likely function as moderator variables; this means that mental health outcomes may be different depending on an individual's level of religious/spiritual involvement. Religion and spirituality have been found to protect against the development of psychological symptoms and to aid recovery and treatment.[42] Below we provide some examples of the role of religion in mental health outcomes and then review two studies directly investigating the role of religion in treatment.

Spirituality was found to relate to treatment outcomes in an outpatient substance misuse program.[6] Higher levels of spirituality before entering a substance misuse treatment predicted better treatment outcome over and above effects due to personality. However, the analyses did not control for scores on the outcome measures at the start of treatment, thus spirituality cannot be said to relate to change that occurred during treatment. In addition, findings that pretreatment scores on measures of religion or spirituality predict treatment outcomes do not directly address whether it would be beneficial for psychological treatments to be modified to target individuals for whom religion or spirituality is particularly important (or unimportant). Below we describe two studies that directly address this question.

Azhar et al.[44] investigated the incremental efficacy of adding religious psychotherapy to a combination of supportive psychotherapy and anxiolytic medications for a sample of religious individuals with generalized anxiety disorder. Half of the participants received the additional component of religious psychotherapy, which consisted of discussions of specific religious issues. Participants who received religious psychotherapy showed greater reductions in anxiety symptoms after treatment. We would like to note, however, that neither supportive psychotherapy nor discussions of religious issues are considered front-line empirically supported treatments (ESTs) for anxiety disorders (e.g., see reference 45 for a discussion of ESTs). Thus, future work is needed to see if supportive psychotherapy plus discussion of religious issues is a better treatment for anxiety disorders in religious individuals than front-line empirically supported treatments such as exposure and cognitive-behavioral therapy (CBT).

Propst and colleagues[46] suggested that the emphasis on personal autonomy and self-efficacy in traditional CBT may not fit with the cultural values of some religious individuals with worldviews centered around dependence on God. They tested whether a religiously framed modification of CBT (RCT) would be more efficacious for self-identified Christian individuals than a standard CBT protocol (NRCT). These researchers also included a pastoral counseling condition (PCT), which contained all of the nonspecific factors of religious counseling without the active components of CBT. The study additionally included a wait-list control. The study also investigated whether nonreligious therapists could implement the religious modification of CBT by including an equal number of religious and nonreligious therapists in both CBT conditions. All participants believed that the treatment program was religious to a certain extent: they were told that some therapists would be explicitly religious, whereas others would not, but that all therapists would be respectful of and encouraging toward their religious beliefs and relationship to God. The religious CBT protocol (RCT) included Christian religious rationales for the procedures, religious arguments to counter irrational thoughts, and religious imagery.

Post-treatment results indicated that participants in RCT reported greater reductions in depressive symptoms and greater improvements in social adjustment and general symptomatology than participants in a waiting list control, whereas patients in standard CBT did not report greater reductions than waiting list control participants. The finding that standard CBT was not better than a wait-list control is not consistent with a robust finding in the literature than CBT is an effective treatment for depression and better than wait-list control (e.g., reference 45). This finding suggests two possibilities: first, that the standard CBT used in this study was not a "full dose" of CBT. This possibility could explain why standard CBT was not better than wait-list control in this sample. It would also suggest that the

RCT may have outperformed standard CBT in this sample because it contained additional "ingredients" of CBT (e.g., rationale) that gave patients a "full dose" of the treatment. In this case, the religious modification may have been more effective because additional content was used, not necessarily because that content was religious in nature. The use of a treatment group with additional nonreligious components was not used, thus this hypothesis was not tested.

Propst and colleagues[46] provided a different interpretation of their findings. They reported that traditional CBT and pastoral counseling performed similarly in this population (though direct statistical tests of this claim were not performed). They suggested that in a religious population, consideration of clients' religious worldviews may be as efficacious as the active ingredients of CBT. Thus, the fact that traditional CBT did not do better than a wait-list control in this sample may be due to differences between religious samples and the samples normally used to test the efficacy of CBT.

Propst and colleagues[46] also reported that at three-month and two-year follow-up, no differences in depressive symptoms were found between the treatment conditions. Thus, the superiority of the religious modification of CBT was not maintained over time. The authors also reported that tests of effects due to therapists' religious orientations indicate that the treatment group showing the greatest reduction in depressive symptoms was the religious modification of CBT conducted by nonreligious therapists. This suggests that modifying a treatment to include religious content is sufficient for therapeutic enhancement – particular therapists are not necessary to implement the treatment. This study suggests that modifying the content of traditional CBT for depression to better match the worldviews of religious clients may be relatively more efficacious for religious clients. However, the lack of a comparison group of nonreligious clients as well as a lack of differences at follow-up precludes drawing conclusions about the efficacy of matching clients to religious or nonreligious treatments based on pretreatment religious beliefs or practices. Additional research is needed to understand whether religious modifications of existing ESTs lead to better treatment outcomes for religious individuals.

COMPREHENSIVE CASE EXAMPLE

Monica was a 30-year-old married woman who presented with symptoms of OCD and depression. During the intake interview, she explained that she was a devout Catholic and that many of her rituals involved prayer. She reported that she married her husband when she was 23 and did not have sex until her wedding night. One year ago Monica had an affair with a man she met through friends. The relationship lasted for about two months, at which point she ended it, as guilt regarding the affair was causing her great distress. She had not told her husband about the affair and many of her rituals involved repenting and spiritual cleansing to "erase the sin of the affair".

During the intake process, Monica was encouraged to explain her religious views, and she expressed great conflict with regard to her religion. She reported that she was raised as a devout Catholic, and that she endorsed the belief that premarital sex is wrong and that having an affair is a sin. Her husband was also a strongly religious individual and she worried that telling him of her affair would not only hurt him emotionally but would cause him to see her as a sinner. She felt that she had no one to talk to about this because all of her friends were also religious and she believed they would condemn her for what she had done. She expressed hope that by praying and repenting daily she could cleanse her soul and make amends for the sin she had committed.

Monica reported spending two to three hours daily engaged in her prayer rituals. She also indicated spending another one to two hours engaged in cleansing rituals, including two showers daily and multiple hand-washings. She additionally reported that she had been feeling very guilty regarding her affair and that having had the affair meant she was a weak person morally. She had difficulty sleeping at night and had lost weight over the past few months. Monica insisted that she was not suicidal, as she believed that suicide was a sin.

Monica and her therapist initially decided to focus on her symptoms of depression, as she indicated that those symptoms were more distressing than her OCD symptoms. The initial treatment plan consisted of IPT role transition to help Monica come to terms with the fact that she could not be a "perfect Catholic" as she had struggled to be for so long. Using the techniques of IPT, Monica's therapist was able to remain nonjudgmental by allowing Monica to talk through her feelings and work on transitioning to a role that was more comfortable for her. In addition, the therapist provided support and understanding when Monica told of her affair so that Monica would not feel judged. Below is a transcript of an example session between Monica and her therapist.

Therapist (T): So, Monica, tell me how you have been feeling since I saw you last.

Monica (M): I've been feeling like such a failure. All my life I have tried to be a perfect Catholic but I'm really not. I had an affair! That is so wrong!

T: It sounds like you are holding yourself to a very high standard. Are all other Catholics perfect?

M: No, I guess not. But I have always tried to be perfect and I just keep failing. I feel like I am not worthy.

T: What are you not worthy of?

M: I'm not worthy of . . . God's love, I guess. And my husband's love too. He made a commitment to be with me and then when I had my affair I just totally abandoned him and abandoned my faith.

T: Was that what you were thinking when you had your affair? That you were abandoning your husband and your faith?

M: No, not really. I think I was just really unhappy with how my relationship with my husband was and I sort of acted impulsively. I really liked this guy and he liked me, he seemed to understand me more than my husband does and that was appealing to me. I didn't think about how it would impact my marriage or my faith until later.

T: So you weren't trying to abandon your husband or your faith.

M: No. But that doesn't really matter, does it? I mean, the bottom line is that I committed a sin whether I meant to or not.

T: Is that really the bottom line? Do your religious traditions mandate that you must never make mistakes or act impulsively?

M: Well, I don't know. I guess it is okay to make mistakes. Maybe if you confess your sins then it will be okay.

T: That makes sense. Because a lot of people make mistakes.

M: Yeah, that's true. I guess everyone makes mistakes sometimes, but not all of them are sins. It's worse when it is a sin. I don't think perfect Catholics ever sin, even by mistake.

T: Really? Perfect Catholics don't sin at all? That's pretty impressive. It must be really hard not to ever sin.

M: Well, if the Lord is really with you, that makes it a lot easier. He helps you so that you don't sin.

T: I see. So let's say, for the moment, that perfect Catholics are people who don't ever sin. What does this mean for you, that you are no longer a perfect Catholic?

M: Well, I . . . I'm not really sure. I feel like a failure. I feel like God is disappointed in me.

T: That must be difficult. A few minutes ago, though, you said that maybe if you confessed it would be okay.

M: Yeah, I keep thinking that I should go to confession but I am really embarrassed. I don't want my priest to know about my affair. I'm afraid that he would look down on me.

T: Really? I thought that priests were supposed to be understanding and to help us to forgive ourselves.

M: Yes, they are, but he's human too!

T: What do you mean by that?

M: He's supposed to be all nice and forgiving because he's a priest but he's also a human and humans judge others.

T: You are right, humans do judge others, but they are also understanding and forgiving. People tend to be especially forgiving when the person who made the mistake is really sorry.

M: And I am really sorry!

T: I know you are. These last few sessions, as you've been telling me about your affair and how you feel about it, has it made you feel better at all?

M: It has, actually. I was really nervous to tell you about it at first but now it is kind of a relief to be able to talk about it.

T: Maybe going to confession would also be a relief?

M: I think so. Maybe it won't be as bad as I think. I mean, I was afraid that you would judge me but I feel like you haven't, so maybe my priest wouldn't judge me either. I had a time of weakness but now I am very sorry about it and I want to do whatever I can to make amends and not ever let this happen again.

At her next appointment, Monica reported that she had gone to confession. She said that it was very difficult for her but she felt that her priest was understanding. However, she continued to report feelings of guilt and distress. The following session, she admitted that she had been considering leaving her husband, but that she also felt leaving the marriage would be another failure on her part. She reported dissatisfaction with the marriage and a desire to experience life on her own. However, these feelings were also causing her great distress as she believed that divorce was wrong and that she had made a lifelong commitment to her husband the day they were married. At this point, treatment switched to Motivational Interviewing[47] so that Monica could explore her feelings of ambivalence regarding her marriage.

After several sessions of Motivational Interviewing, Monica decided that it was very important to her to remain in her marriage and work on improving it. She generated a list of things that she and her husband could do to improve their relationship. Her symptoms of depression began to decrease but she still reported significant feelings of guilt regarding her affair. Treatment at this time switched back to IPT role transition and several sessions were spent discussing what makes a "perfect Catholic" and what makes a "good Catholic." Monica was able to recognize that being a "good Catholic" might be enough to make her feel happy and that making mistakes is part of being human. As her symptoms of depression continued to decrease, Monica found that her symptoms of OCD also began to decrease.

In later sessions, exposure with response prevention was used to help Monica further reduce the time spent on her ritualized behaviors that stemmed from her OCD diagnosis. She maintained that it was still important to her that she pray daily but she was able to reduce her amount of time spent in prayer to 30 minutes. She was also able to eliminate all of her cleansing rituals. After the final sessions spent discussing the gains Monica had made and suggestions to help her in the future, therapy was terminated, in keeping with our clinic's practice of continuing treatment for 8–12 sessions following symptom remission.

By being nonjudgmental and open, the therapist was able to create an environment in which Monica felt comfortable discussing her affair as well as her thoughts regarding divorce. In particular, Monica's fears of being judged were alleviated by the therapist's nonjudgmental stance. The therapist was able to remain impartial, offering no advice regarding whether or not Monica should divorce her husband, allowing Monica to come to a decision herself. Using the techniques of Motivational Interviewing, the therapist simply encouraged Monica to talk through her reasons for and against divorce until she was able to make a decision. When they turned to the symptoms of OCD, the therapist allowed Monica to set her own goals regarding the amount of prayer that she was comfortable engaging in and the therapist simply helped Monica to achieve her goals. They worked on slowly confining prayer to a certain time of day and reducing the amount of time spent on prayer until Monica reached her goal of 30 minutes per day. The therapist did not force Monica to eliminate prayer completely, as Monica emphasized that it was important to her to spend some time praying each day.

CONCLUSIONS AND FUTURE DIRECTIONS

Two studies have suggested that modifications of existing treatments to include religious components may be efficacious for religious individuals.[44,46] However, neither of these studies allows for inferences about the causal mechanisms contributing to the efficacy of the religious components of treatment. Therefore, it is difficult to generalize these results to other treatments in terms of suggesting the form of potential treatment modifications. Propst and colleagues[46] found that a modification of traditional CBT based on Beck and colleagues'[48] model was effective for individuals who identify as Christian. However, it is unclear to what extent similar modifications in terms of rationale for treatment would be incrementally useful for the type of CBT presented in this chapter. To address this issue, future research investigating the efficacy of CBASP for highly religious and spiritual individuals is needed as well as research investigating potentially differential mechanisms of treatment effects or client experiences in CBT based on Beck and colleagues'[48] framework compared with CBASP.

In closing, Richards and Bergin[4] call for an increase in spiritual sensitivity and competency among mental health professionals. We suggested that treatments which use clients' personal goals and formulations of success as the framework for intervention may be especially acceptable to – and helpful for – individuals with strongly held religious and spiritual beliefs. Future research specifically addressing this hypothesis is needed before strong recommendations can be made; however, consistent with the need for culture-specific expertise, we suggest (with an air of hopeful caution) that spiritual sensitivity and competency may be increased (at least in part) by familiarization with common religious/spiritual beliefs and practices as well as familiarization with the techniques of a spiritually sensitive treatment.

CHAPTER 6

The Assessment, Diagnosis, and Treatment of Psychiatric Disorders in Children and Families from Diverse Backgrounds

Kendra R Tannenbaum, Carla Counts-Allan, Lara J Jakobsons, and Karla K Repper

Behavioral parent training is one of the most widely used interventions for children with externalizing problem behaviors. This type of treatment has emerged as an empirically supported intervention for this population, and reviews have consistently demonstrated the efficacy of behavioral management techniques in reducing problem behaviors.[1,2] A number of studies, however, have indicated that these techniques are not successful for all families, and that characteristics of the parent, child, and environment affect treatment outcome.[3,4] Specifically, ethnic diversity, resource availability/socioeconomic status (SES), and family structure (e.g., single parent families, grandparent or other legal guardian as primary caregiver, multiple caregivers in multiple households) may moderate treatment effects. These variables are important for clinicians to consider when providing treatment to a family, as they likely play a role in the assessment, diagnosis, and treatment of problematic externalizing behaviors. In fact, assessment tools and intervention techniques may need to be modified to enhance the success of a parent training program.

Our goal in writing this chapter is to increase clinicians' awareness of variables such as ethnic diversity, resource availability/SES, and family structure, and the role they may play in the assessment, diagnosis, and treatment of problematic childhood externalizing behaviors. The case examples presented throughout the chapter reflect scenarios that we have directly observed in our community-based outpatient clinic. Specifically, these examples focus on children and adolescents who have been diagnosed with attention-deficit hyperactivity disorder (ADHD), oppositional defiant disorder (ODD), and/or conduct disorder. Treatment in our clinic for these disorders emphasizes empirically supported techniques such as positive reinforcement, involvement in and monitoring of children's activities, consistency, use of time-out as a punishment technique, and use of a token economy.[5,6] When assessing, diagnosing, and treating externalizing problem behaviors, clinicians need to be mindful of the variables that may affect treatment outcome, and they may need to modify their expectations based on the characteristics of the family. Behavioral parent training will ultimately be most effective if clinicians develop expertise in working with diverse families. Skills such as scientific mindedness[7] (i.e., forming and testing hypotheses about families from diverse backgrounds) and dynamic sizing[7] (i.e., knowing when it is appropriate to apply knowledge of a family's culture to the child's behavior) will allow clinicians to appreciate and effectively work with families from diverse backgrounds.

CLINICAL OBSERVATIONS
Assessment

Diversity plays an important role in the assessment of child behavior problems. In particular, clinicians make diagnostic decisions for children based on how their behavior is perceived by adults. Each adult has a unique perspective on the presenting problem, and many variables affect the lens through which child behavior is viewed and determined to be problematic. These variables include family structure, culture, SES, and parenting style. For example, a single mother and her 8-year-old son, Jake, came to our clinic to receive parent training after receiving a referral from Jake's school for oppositional and aggressive behavior. Jake's mother admitted to feeling stressed and guilty with regard to her parenting ability and life choices. More specifically, she believed that many of Jake's externalizing behaviors could be attributed to an underlying anxiety disorder. Further, she suggested that these behaviors were the result of Jake witnessing several occasions during which she was physically abused by Jake's father. Jake's mother and teachers seemed to examine his behavior through different lenses, causing problems in their communication. Jake tended to be frustrated by tasks that required sustained mental effort and left the classroom without permission to avoid these tasks. He also frequently ran outside the house when his mother asked him to complete his household chores. Although the behavior across the settings was similar, Jake's mother thought that he was responding to anxiety stemming from a performance fear. In contrast, the school urged his mother to have Jake examined for stimulant medication for ADHD to help him concentrate for longer periods of time. Consequently, the interaction between school and home was often strained, causing both parties to be ignorant about behavior occurring across both settings.

Fortunately, Jake's clinician took a scientifically minded approach to the assessment process and formed two hypotheses about his behavioral presentation:

- Jake's externalizing behaviors may stem from an attention disorder
- Jake's externalizing behaviors may stem from an underlying anxiety disorder.

As a result, a thorough assessment was necessary in order to test these two hypotheses. Several rating scales that have demonstrated reliability and validity (i.e., Conners Rating Scales-Revised;[8] ADHD Rating Scale-IV;[9] Child Behavior Checklist [CBCL][10]) were completed by Jake's mother and teacher, and his profile suggested the presence of ADHD with subthreshold social and separation anxiety symptomatology. During the feedback session, Jake's mother became frustrated mostly because she had previously been given the diagnosis of ADHD for Jake in other clinical settings and did not feel it was accurate. In addition, she had previously tried behavioral management techniques with little success, and felt that the treatment failure reflected misdiagnosis. In general, she appeared overwhelmed regarding her ability to manage Jake's ADHD symptoms, possibly because she was a single parent with a full-time job. Rather, she stressed that his externalizing behavior was in response to fears of separation and often occurred during the presence of panic attacks endorsed as "temper tantrums" on behavioral rating scales. Jake's mother appeared to be more comfortable with anxiety diagnoses and expressed that he just needed more confidence to move beyond his separation anxiety. Moreover, she felt that clinicians, in general, overdiagnose ADHD and suggested that it was due to a "medication agenda". An open and respectful conversation about the causes of Jake's behaviors, and a discussion about the difference in perspectives that existed between Jake's teacher and Jake's mother helped the clinician accurately assess Jake's behaviors and respect his mother's concerns. A diagnosis of ADHD was made, and the clinician used her dynamic sizing skills[7] to appropriately acknowledge that the mother's single-parent status and overall level of stress was contributing to Jake's symptomatology. As such, the clinician spent several sessions helping Jake's mother cope with her single-parent status and discussed ways to modify her hectic lifestyle.

There are many other family and diversity variables that should be taken into consideration during an assessment. It is imperative that clinicians understand the child's family structure in order to pursue the most accurate assessment information possible. In some cultures, children spend a great amount of time with extended family members, and those family members may be responsible for taking care of young children while the parents work. Clinicians often rely on parental reports of child behavior; however, validity can be increased through the collection of assessment data from others who spend significant amounts of time with the child. For example, a mother sought services for her 6-year-old daughter, Alisha, who was demonstrating oppositional behaviors. Alisha's grandmother provided childcare to her and her siblings after school because Alisha's mother had two jobs to support the family. The clinician decided that it would be valuable to obtain assessment information from *both* the grandmother and the mother because Alisha spent several hours with the grandmother every day. Failure to obtain assessment ratings from the grandparent may have interfered with the clinician's ability to establish a clear picture of Alisha's behavior. In general, clinicians should develop dynamic sizing skills[7] (e.g., ability to know when it is necessary to deviate from a traditional protocol that relies primarily on mother's report) and employ them in the appropriate situations.

Relatedly, biological parents are occasionally unable to care for their children, and responsibility may be entrusted to a member of the extended family. For example, a woman and her 10-year-old nephew, Aaron, presented at our clinic for the treatment of ADHD. The woman was caring for her nephew because his parents had been recently incarcerated. In this case, it was likely that the new caretakers would have been unable to report the child's history (e.g., developmental milestones, onset of problem behavior, etc.) with confidence. Thus, it is important for clinicians to consider the effect this may have on the accuracy of assessment information and attempt to obtain information from the biological parents to receive as much information as possible.

In addition, attitudes about normal child development and problem behavior may differ depending on the background of the rater. Culture greatly influences both what is considered normative and maladaptive. If clinicians have a greater understanding of the family's culture, they may be able to make better sense of discrepancies between raters (e.g., parents and teachers). Culture-specific expertise[7] may lead to the application of helpful interventions, as well as facilitate communication between the clinician, the child's family, and the child's school. For example, an Asian American family came to the clinic seeking services for their 13-year-old son, Hao, who was exhibiting oppositional behavior. After Hao's parents and teachers completed reliable behavioral rating scales, it became clear to the clinician that they viewed his behavior from different lenses. Hao's family moved to the United States when he was an infant. Relative to Hao's teachers, his parents had little information about normative child development in the United States. In particular, his parents rated Hao as highly oppositional, whereas his teachers' ratings placed him in the "normal" range on all of the rating scales. More specifically, Hao's parents expressed dissatisfaction with his apparent disregard for the family's traditional beliefs. Knowledge about the family's background made it possible to assess the effect of culture on ratings. As a result, Hao's parents were relieved to know that his behavior was typical by American standards, but they continued to express desire for Hao to behave in a manner more consistent with Asian standards. The clinician then initiated a discussion with the family about normative behaviors in the United States but stressed that the family should feel free to discuss their cultural values throughout the treatment process to make the clinician more aware of their specific behavioral goals for Hao.

Parenting style is also an important aspect of diversity to consider with regard to assessment practices. For example, a key first step in the development of behavioral treatment strategies is establishing antecedents and consequences to behavior. Sometimes parents are afraid to disclose information about discipline practices, perhaps in an attempt to avoid negative evaluation by the clinician. For example, a mother sought parent training for help in dealing with her 8-year-old son's problems with oppositional behavior. Initially, she was unwilling to disclose her discipline practices because she feared that the clinician would not approve of the corporal punishment techniques she used. Thus, it is crucial for clinicians to establish a neutral, nonjudgmental stance from the first interaction with a family, while also explaining their ethical duty to report suspected abuse. Failure to be supportive and understanding may compromise rapport and disclosure on behalf of the family, leading to an incomplete assessment.

In conclusion, children are a part of their family system, and the assessment of their behavior must occur within that system. In order for clinicians to receive an accurate and complete representation of the child's current level of functioning, an open and trusting relationship between the clinician and the child's family must be established. Clinicians should have a firm understanding of the family structure, culture, parenting style, and family history to fully consider the lens through which child behavior is viewed. Moreover, culturally competent clinicians know when it is appropriate to apply knowledge of a particular family's culture to the assessment process.[7]

Diagnosis

Family-system diversity also plays an important role with regard to diagnosis. Unfortunately, clinicians are not immune to common stereotypes, and neither are the child's caretakers or the school in which the child functions. Beliefs in stereotypes, whether conscious or not, may lead to incorrect diagnosis and misunderstandings between the clinician and the child's caretakers. These beliefs may stem from popular culture (e.g., music videos, television advertisements), and if strongly believed, they may cause clinicians to fail to attend to relevant diagnostic information. Although clinicians are not immune to stereotypes, mindfulness and awareness of their beliefs may help minimize diagnostic errors. Competent clinicians possess knowledge of their own general views, as well as specific knowledge about diverse families. Also, competent clinicians possess dynamic sizing skills and know when it is appropriate to make valid generalizations from their initial beliefs.[7]

It is extremely important that clinicians tailor diagnostic feedback to the family. Different caregivers will have different reactions to hearing that their child meets diagnostic criteria for a particular disorder. Psychoeducation (i.e., presentation of relevant information about psychological disorders, possible causes, course, and treatment) is a crucial component of the feedback session. Specifically, clinicians will be able to better assist the family if they have an understanding of how caretakers are likely to interpret the diagnosis. Moreover, feedback should be tailored to the role of the caretaker, such that a single mother with full custody of her child may receive information that is different from information received by a father who has custody of the child on alternate weekends. In other words, when both parents are not living together, it may be necessary to spend a lot of time discussing the need for consistency across both households; in contrast, if only the mother is present, it may be important to focus discussion on communication between school and home.

An African American child, Thomas, and his grandmother presented at our clinic to gain a deeper understanding of why Thomas' grades were declining in third grade. Thomas had moved the summer before third grade and was having difficulty adjusting to his new school. His grandmother believed that he was the victim of discrimination on the part of his new teacher and school administration. In addition, she was concerned that he was the only African American child in his classroom and one of the few minorities within the elementary school. As a result, she believed his minority status contributed to his poor grades and frequent referrals to the principal's office because he had done well the previous year in a predominately African American elementary school. Thomas' grandmother also mentioned that his teacher stated that he "wasn't third grade material" and should repeat third grade. Thomas' grandmother was understandably upset about the situation, and one of her goals for the assessment was to "prove the school wrong". This desire may have caused her to underreport Thomas' problems on behavioral rating scales, as there was a clear mismatch between her ratings and the teacher's ratings. This mismatch between raters complicated the establishment of a clear diagnostic picture.

Thomas' clinician took a scientifically minded approach to the diagnostic process to determine whether his poor grades and referrals to the principal's office were a result of discrimination on the part of his school or an underlying behavior disorder. Rather than simply relying on the ratings completed by Thomas' grandmother, the clinician also utilized a semi-structured clinical interview that allowed his grandmother to be more open. In fact, Thomas' grandmother was more willing to disclose problem behavior during the structured clinical interview. Specifically, Thomas' grandmother stated that she did not like the rating scales because they did not allow her to explain the context in which Thomas' behavior problems occurred. Therefore, information collected from the interview was more consistent with the teacher ratings of Thomas' behavior and was weighed more heavily in the establishment of a diagnosis.

On examination of the information provided by Thomas' grandmother and teachers, he met diagnostic criteria for ADHD. His grandmother admitted that she was nervous about how the school would interpret the diagnosis and was worried that he would be labeled as a "problem child". In addition, she was suspicious of psychostimulant medication and expressed a desire to continue using herbal supplements to control his hyperactivity. However, when given extensive psychoeducational information regarding the prevalence of ADHD and the efficacy of medication as a frontline treatment for ADHD, she became relieved. In short, Thomas' grandmother did not initially believe the diagnosis was correct because she thought he was the victim of discrimination; however, after a frank discussion about her concerns, as well as psychoeducation about the symptoms of ADHD, she ultimately expressed gratitude for "hanging in there" with her throughout the diagnostic process.

Treatment

When treating diverse families, a variety of unique and challenging clinical issues may present themselves. For instance, in most parent training programs, the term "parents" typically refers to the mother. However, in more diverse families, parent training may need to be modified based on who is actually implementing the treatment. Competent clinicians use their dynamic sizing skills to know when it is appropriate to apply knowledge of the family structure to the child's behavior.[7] Ultimately, this may require the clinician to deviate from the standard treatment protocol. For example, a Latino client in his mid-twenties, Ramón, sought parent training for his son, Alex, who was demonstrating oppositional behaviors. Ramón and his wife held more traditional roles often found in some Latino cultures, and the child rearing responsibilities primarily fell on his wife. However, his wife was incarcerated several months before Ramón sought services, which left him in the primary parenting role.

During therapy, a unique issue became apparent in that Ramón appeared notably uncomfortable with the parenting role and viewed his 6-year-old son more as a "playmate" than his child. Specifically, Ramón demonstrated difficulty setting rules and boundaries which were integral to the implementation of a home token economy to decrease Alex's oppositional behavior. A home token economy is a program where tokens and praise are given to the child following the absence of a problematic behavior or the presence of an appropriate behavior. The tokens reinforce the child for displaying appropriate behaviors and are then exchanged for rewards. In particular, Ramón showed difficulty in providing firm commands to his son and frequently did not follow through on the commands. It became evident to both the clinician and Ramón that he had limited knowledge of childrearing practices because the parenting role previously fell in his wife's domain. As a result, Ramón's lack of influence over his son weakened his ability to implement and enforce the token system. In this instance, it was necessary for the clinician to teach the father about child development and the role of the parent, emphasizing the need for consistency and authority. If Ramón's therapist had not possessed these dynamic sizing skills and cultural expertise,[7] the treatment would have been less likely to have effective. In addition, the clinician capitalized on Ramón's strengths, such as his affection and playfulness towards Alex. Likewise, Ramón was encouraged to use play and affection to reinforce appropriate behavior, and the clinician praised Ramón in these instances.

Another challenge in the treatment of diverse families may be evident when two parents live in the same household and only one of them participates in treatment. Ideally, consistency would be increased if one parent shared and taught the techniques to the other parent. However, this may not always be possible. For example, a client, Joshua, sought parent training for his teenage son. His wife did not participate in therapy because she thought it implied that she was not a "good mother." At first, Joshua attempted to teach her the parenting skills. She initially responded and they established the house rules and punishments together. Whereas Joshua maintained consistency fairly well, his wife showed difficulty enforcing the rules (e.g., "caving in" and not grounding the son after he violated a rule). In turn, this created inconsistency in parenting and tension between the couple. As a result, Joshua realized that the implementation of the parenting skills by both of them was not effective. The differing views on parenting held by Joshua and his wife, as well as other problems in their marriage, ultimately led to a divorce. Following the divorce, they shared custody of their son. When he stayed with his father, the son understood that his father's rules would remain consistent, which ultimately led to an increase in the son's compliance. Although this example may seem a bit drastic, it underscores the importance of maintaining consistency between parents in a household.

In some cultures, children spend larger amounts of time with extended family members, which can affect treatment. For instance, some African American and Hispanic/Latino families may rely heavily on extended family and neighbors to help care for their children. Likely, this is attributable to these cultures' value of "family" and of interdependence. Reliance on extended family may also be the result of limited resources to pay for childcare or a hectic work schedule. However, the children's relatives may not be directly involved in the therapy process, which could impact treatment outcome by limiting consistency in child rearing. For example, if a child's grandmother takes care of him during the week and he lives with his parents during the weekend, the benefits of therapy may be enhanced by involving both sets of caretakers in parent training. Another option would be for the parents to share and teach the specific techniques to the grandmother. A clinician who possesses culture-specific expertise and dynamic sizing skills understands the importance of extended families in some cultures and uses this knowledge to modify the standard treatment protocol. Overall, this example illustrates the need for consistency in parenting, which becomes even more important when children are cared for by extended family members.

In comparison with large and extended families, some families are not intact, which can present unique challenges. In particular, consistency during the implementation of discipline and reinforcement may become difficult, especially if the child regularly moves between different homes. For example, a disabled client sought parent training for her three grandsons (of whom she held legal guardianship). The children's father lived several houses away from the grandmother and visited his sons daily. Their mother lived across town with her boyfriend and took care of the children during weekends. In short, the children were often moved between the three homes, and each household had distinct rules. As a result, the children's behavior problems and negative interactions among family members increased due to a lack of consistency. When the children's father joined the parent training, it was the first time that the father and grandmother had worked together on implementing consistent parenting skills. Through the parent training, the father and grandmother agreed on rules that would be enforced and gradually increased positive interactions with the children.

Although the children's mother was not involved in the parent training (which complicated treatment in that it decreased the consistency of the techniques), substantial gains were still observed. Specifically, on returning to the grandmother's household after visiting their mother, the children's behavior problems would occasionally increase. However, this occurred sporadically, and she observed that the behavior problems would decrease again within a few hours. This appeared to occur because the grandmother and father were able to maintain consistency within their households. The children realized that whenever they returned to their father or grandmother, the same rules and expectations held as prior to their visitation with their mother. Overall, this example illustrates that despite the lack of one caregiver's participation in treatment, children's behavior problems in other households can decrease through the implementation of consistent parenting by other caregivers.

Many diverse families may have limited financial resources, which may impact the ability to set up a token economy system that provides material reinforcements. Praise and attention, in the absence of material reinforcement, are often sufficient in shaping children's behavior. Therefore, it is possible for families of all socioeconomic backgrounds to implement token economy systems using natural reinforcement. For example, a client who was unemployed sought parent training for her granddaughter, Allison. Initially, she expressed doubt regarding the feasibility of a point system that is traditionally based on material reinforcement. As a result, the client and her clinician brainstormed alternative and less costly motivators, such as stickers and small snacks. In particular, verbal and nonverbal reinforcement, such as praise, attention, affection, and inexpensive activities were emphasized and became very important motivators for increasing positive behaviors in Allison. In addition, activities such as reading a story to her at bedtime as well as free activities in the community, such as trips to the zoo and walks in the park, proved to be highly effective reinforcement. Thus, inexpensive and creative reinforcements are as powerful as material rewards and are available for clients who have limited financial resources. Although most behavioral parent training programs rely in part on material reinforcements, culturally competent clinicians devise alternative methods of reinforcement when the family's culture dictates that this is necessary.

THE CURRENT STATE OF THE LITERATURE
Assessment and Diagnosis

As discussed earlier, diversity affects the lens through which child behavior is viewed by parents, teachers, and diagnosticians, creating a strong need for multi-method, multi-informant assessment techniques. Clinicians should aim to gather information from as many different sources as possible, with a special focus on the child's caretakers (e.g., parents, grandparents, aunts, uncles) and teachers. Similarly, the multi-informant strategy will be strengthened if multi-method strategies are used as well, as individuals from different cultural backgrounds may respond more favorably to one method than another (e.g., Thomas' grandmother was more forthcoming using structured interview when compared to ratings scales). The following section attempts to elucidate additional considerations regarding how diversity affects assessment and diagnosis in light of the current scientific literature.

Some assessment instruments may not be appropriate or relevant to various cultural groups. In fact, many instruments have been developed, standardized, and normed almost exclusively with middle to upper class European American samples.[11] The development, standardization, and normative processes strongly influence the appropriate use of the instrument, and research has demonstrated some problems in the application of instruments to minority samples. For example, the CBCL[10] has been shown to lack adequate coverage of items for clinically relevant behavior in a sample of African American children.[12]

Additional research on the CBCL by Weisz et al.[13] further lends support to cautious use of the measure in ethnic and racial minority groups. Specifically, the syndrome structure of clinic-referred children in the United States and Thailand were compared and great differences were found across narrowband measures of behavior (i.e., more specific groups of behaviors, such as aggression, anxiety, sexual problems). However, the broadband measures of behavior (i.e. broader groupings of behavior, such as externalizing and internalizing behavior) were more promising and demonstrated moderate agreement between countries. Weisz et al.[13] suggested that clinicians use caution with measures such as the CBCL because the lens through which child behavior is viewed and rated is dependent on culture and societal norms. These perceived differences in syndrome structure likely affect the way children with diverse backgrounds are diagnosed in the United States. Thus, the CBCL may have differential validity and utility in various ethnic groups, which should be considered in the diagnostic process. When using these measures with culturally diverse families, clinicians should take a scientific-minded approach and develop and test hypotheses about the pattern of results. In addition, knowledge of the cultural group may help the clinician understand the results, as well as minimize their biases in interpretation.[7]

Diversity in family structure should also be taken into consideration when formulating goals and assessing treatment success or failure. Family structure is relevant because research has shown that single-parent status is predictive of more negative behaviors and greater child deviance.[4] Consequently, clinicians should consider this information when a single parent and child present for treatment, especially during the case conceptualization process and the development of appropriate goals and time frames. Further, it may take longer for children of single-parent homes to show improvement than children within intact families. Webster-Stratton and Hammond[4] concluded that there may be different predictors of success depending on the treatment goal that has been selected, and they suggest that parent training focus on the specific needs of each family. Dynamic sizing skills are necessary for the clinician to determine when it is appropriate to deviate from the standard assessment and treatment protocol based on the family structure.[7] Failure to tailor assessment and treatment to each family's needs may contribute to treatment failure.

Parenting style is another important consideration because it affects the lens through which behavior is evaluated during the assessment process, which ultimately has implications for diagnosis as well. Moreover, parenting styles that appear to be maladaptive in some contexts may prove to be adaptive in other contexts.[14] For example, Pinderhughes *et al.*[15] showed that African American parents reported higher levels of harsh discipline. Harsh discipline may serve as a protective factor for inner-city youth, such that harsher parenting may decrease the amount of risk factors to which children are exposed.[16] Alternatively, higher levels of harsh discipline may be explained by the relative weight given to the development of different child competencies (e.g., independence) for parents in low SES communities compared with those in high SES communities (e.g., compliance).[17] For example, low SES parents may believe more strongly in the value of spanking as a way to develop emotional independence and self-sufficiency in their children, which are important goals for inner-city youth. On the other hand, parents in higher SES communities may value different competencies for their children and may appreciate different discipline strategies to help their children develop these competencies. Simply stated, harsher discipline and parenting may be somewhat adaptive depending on the child's culture and environment. Competent clinicians possess culture-specific expertise and attempt to understand the function of parenting style across different cultures in order to conduct a thorough assessment and arrive at the most appropriate diagnosis.[7]

Some families may feel a significant amount of shame regarding their child's problem behavior or may distrust mental health professionals. This should be addressed in the first meeting with the family to facilitate honest communication between the clinician and caretakers. For example, Yao[18] suggested that Asian American families may feel uncomfortable sharing their innermost feelings with strangers. Consequently, it is the responsibility of the clinician to address this possibility with the family on the first meeting, with a goal of normalizing the experience so that the lines of communication are opened. Clinicians who lack culture-specific expertise may not understand why some parents are less forthcoming in their disclosure of child behavior problems. Culturally competent clinicians also attempt to understand the cultural values of each family in order to foster feelings of trust. Perhaps the clinician could ask questions related to how child misbehavior is traditionally handled or what the ideal child looks like within the parent's culture, rather than ignore cultural differences.

Forehand and Kotchick[11] stress the importance of talking about parental concerns related to acculturation in parent training. For instance, if a parent fears that parent training will sculpt their child's behavior into that which is valued by majority cultures, they may be concerned about the effect the treatment will have on their family values. Clinicians should make every attempt to understand the parent's perspective and fears, with the ultimate goal of making it clear that their experience is normal and fears will be taken seriously by the clinician. In the end, it will be important for clinicians to help the family problem solve and think through solutions to their concerns.

Careful consideration should be taken in the process of identifying clinically relevant child behaviors because what constitutes problematic behavior may change for various ethnic groups. Clinicians who possess culture-specific expertise understand that noncompliance and aggression are often viewed as problematic in

Caucasian samples, but these behaviors may be viewed as protective in low SES urban areas.[17] Additionally, behavior problems and psychological disorders may be perceived to have different structures in different cultures.[13]

Treatment

The treatment implications of ethnicity, resource availability/SES, and family structure have been the focus of many behavioral parent training studies over the past decade. For instance, high levels of stress are associated with poverty,[19] making SES an important variable to consider in the treatment process. In addition, the high rates of therapy dropout among minorities and single-parent families[20,21] underscore the necessity of understanding the role these variables may play in the treatment process. To understand the role ethnicity might play in the treatment process, it is important to examine variations in parenting practice based on cultural values and ethnicity. Culture-specific expertise will aid clinicians in translating standard behavioral parent training programs into more culturally consistent strategies.[7] The following descriptions of cultural variation in parenting practices do not take into account the diversity within each cultural group. As such, readers are cautioned against making sweeping generalizations about particular ethnic groups.

The dominant culture in the United States emphasizes the Western values of independence and autonomy and is generally oriented toward competition and action (i.e., doing rather than being). In addition, nuclear families rather than extended families are the norm in this culture.[14] Treatment programs are often developed with middle class, European American families in mind. Therefore, the dominant culture has set the "norms" for parenting, creating a deficit model in which cultural differences in parenting practices may be judged as deviant.[11]

The African American culture values the extended family, and mothers often see their children as belonging to a group rather than the nuclear family. As such, parenting is seen as a communal task, with siblings, relatives, and neighbors often caring for and disciplining children.[11,14] Discipline tends to be relatively harsh in African American families compared with European American families. Although many families utilize harsh parenting techniques only occasionally, the prevalence rates are highest among African American and low SES parents.[22] Historically, African American families have used physical punishment as a means to discourage emotional dependency and encourage independence and self-reliance.[17] Religion is also an important factor in African American culture, with the church often providing guidance and support for families.[11,14]

Hispanic/Latino cultures value family loyalty and reliance on extended family for child rearing. The family may include parents, siblings, grandparents, other relatives, and even Godparents and honorary family members.[14] Further, the roles of women and men are often traditional, resulting in the child rearing responsibilities primarily falling on the mother. Hispanic/Latino parents tend to be more permissive and relaxed in their discipline; however, loyalty to the family and obedience to the father is expected of all children.[11,14]

Asian cultures generally value the extended family, and grandparents or other relatives often live in the home or nearby. Although there is a strong expectation for children to obey and respect all elders, the structure of the family is generally patriarchal, with the most respect and obedience given to the oldest male.[14] Success and hard work are particularly valued by Asians, with a strong emphasis on education.[11,14] Discipline in Asian families is often verbally harsh and can involve name-calling and shaming.[14]

Although we are presenting data on African Americans, Hispanic/Latinos, and Asians, these three groups do not constitute all minority groups in the United States. Rather, we are providing specific information about these groups because they constitute three of the largest ethnic and racial minority groups in the United States. Although many of the values of the ethnic minority cultures in the United States are different than the values of the mainstream American culture, most treatment programs were developed using samples of individuals who identify with more mainstream values. It is therefore important for clinicians to understand the values of different cultures and how these values may impact behavioral parent training techniques. With the extended family being the norm for many African American, Hispanic/Latino, and Asian families, many people are encouraged to discipline and care for children.[14] This trend has implications for the treatment of behavior problems, where inconsistent discipline is associated with oppositional and defiant behavior problems.[23,24] As more people are involved in the child rearing process, the risk of inconsistent parenting practices increases. It is also more difficult to implement treatment when multiple caregivers are involved in the process. For instance, as women are often the primary caregivers in Hispanic/Latino families,[14] men may be less likely to participate in treatment, which may also lead to problems with consistency. In addition, ideas of discipline tend to be harsher in African American and Asian families, resulting in potential problems accepting certain parenting techniques, such as time-out and reinforcement of compliance.[11,25] Overall, these cultural differences highlight the importance of considering cultural values when implementing behavioral parent training.

The empirical research on how these cultural differences may affect behavioral parent training is limited. However, despite differences in parenting and family structure across different cultural groups, several studies have found no difference in treatment outcome between Caucasian families and families from ethnic and racial minority groups. For example, Capage et al.[26] provided a 14-week parent training program and found no differences in treatment outcome between African American and Caucasian children (mean age 64 months). In another study, similar results were found with African American, Asian American, Hispanic/Latino and Caucasian children (mean age 56 months).[27] Nevertheless, given the lack of research in this area, the assertion that treatments do not differ culturally is necessarily tentative. Clearly, more studies are needed to compare the efficacy of behavioral parent training in minority families with families from the mainstream cultures, and examine potential cultural variables that may influence parent training techniques. Until further research is conducted, clinicians should take a scientifically minded approach to the treatment of minority families and use their dynamic sizing skills to know when it is appropriate to individualize treatment protocols.

Low SES is another factor that has been found to affect parenting practices. Regardless of ethnicity or age of the child, mothers living in poverty are less likely to communicate effectively with their children, show affection toward their children, and monitor their children, compared with mothers who do not live in poverty.[28] Parents living in poverty are also more likely to use harsh discipline,[15] experience greater levels of stress, and experience decreased levels of support.[19] Overall, these effects are robust across all ethnic groups studied.

In addition to playing a role in parenting practices, SES also affects treatment outcome. Specifically, low SES families are more likely to drop out of behavioral parent training[29] and experience less favorable outcomes at the time of termination.[4,30,31] The negative association between low SES and child improvement may result from a lack of resource availability in low SES families relative to the level of resources often afforded to higher SES families.[32] Limited resources may also diminish the feasibility of implementing techniques commonly taught in behavioral parent training. In one study, low-income African American parents rated time-out procedures as less acceptable than physical punishment.[33] According to the authors of the study, implementation of time-out was hypothesized to be more difficult because of the lack of space in the home. The struggle to meet the daily needs of the family may have also interfered with the implementation of time-consuming methods of punishment, such as time-out. In addition, poverty also limits parents' ability to provide concrete reinforcers and privileges.[28] When treating low SES families, it is imperative for clinicians to be aware of and address the influences of poverty on the success of behavioral parent training. Dynamic sizing skills afford the clinician the ability to know when it is necessary to modify the parent training techniques, such as suggesting alternative consequences if time-out is not feasible or spending extra time identifying affordable reinforcers.[34]

The structure of families in the United States is quite diverse, with children living in a variety of environments such as two-parent households, single-parent households, more than one household (i.e. divorced parents), or with a legal guardian. In particular, single-parent families are more likely to drop out of parent training and present some unique challenges to the clinician.[20] Single-parent families are typically headed by a female, with only 10% of single-parent families headed by a male.[35] Although clinicians tend to think of mothers as the primary parent in behavioral parent training, fathers are also involved in this process, particularly when the father has primary custody of the child.

Although it has not been systematically studied, some researchers have suggested that fathers may have less knowledge about child development, less experience with child care, fewer supports available to assist them with parenting, and more discomfort in the role of primary caregiver.[36,37] These characteristics of fathers likely impact the father–child relationship. Scientifically minded clinicians will test these hypotheses in creative ways during the treatment process and modify the standard treatment protocol as necessary to address the differences in parenting between mothers and fathers.[7] However, fathers may also bring unique qualities to the parent–child interaction that should be reinforced during treatment, such as a sense of security, stimulating play, and a different type of affection than mothers.[36] Although there may be differences in fathers' interactions with their children, research has shown that fathers who undergo behavioral parent training can successfully acquire parenting skills that lead to a reduction in noncompliant behavior.[38,39] In addition, parent training can provide an opportunity to increase fathers' perceptions of parental competence and involvement with their child.[40]

Family structure is increasingly changing across all ethnicities and races, insofar as grandparents are beginning to take a more central parenting role. This particular family structure often results from some type of dysfunction with the parents, such as drug use, incarceration, homelessness, or illness.[41] Taking on the role of primary caregiver as a grandparent often changes the timing of important milestones, such as retirement and freedom from costs associated with caring for a child.[42] Several studies have also found increased levels of poor health and depression in caregiving grandparents of several races and ethnicities, including African American grandparents,[43] Caucasian grandparents,[41,44] and Hispanic/Latino grandparents.[45] Caring for a child as a grandparent is also associated with limitations in daily living, such as caring for personal needs, doing daily tasks, exercising, and resting.[43,44] Interventions for grandparents with behavior disordered grandchildren should incorporate strategies that address the added stressors grandparents may experience when caring for a child. Dynamic sizing skills allow culturally competent clinicians to know when the stressors associated with caring for a child as a grandparent are affecting the child's behavior and treatment process.[7] In this case, culturally competent clinicians could accommodate the treatment process by targeting the problems experienced by the grandparent and emphasizing the rewards of being a grandparent, such as feelings of gratification, devotion, satisfaction, and pride.[43,45]

In addition to family structure, clinicians need to remember that children exist within larger systems, with their families representing just one part of the system. Multisystemic treatment approaches, such as Multisystemic Therapy[46] and Functional Family Therapy,[47] conceptualize clinical problems in terms of the functions they serve within the system. These treatment approaches have demonstrated efficacy across many treatment outcome studies, particularly for children and adolescents with chronic and severe behavior problems.[48,49]

In conclusion, diversity plays a role in many aspects of assessment, diagnosis, and treatment of children with problem behaviors. Culturally competent clinicians possess scientific mindedness, dynamic sizing skills, and culture-specific expertise.[7] Proficiency in these three characteristics may allow clinicians to better assist families from diverse backgrounds and therefore demonstrate better treatment outcomes.

COMPREHENSIVE CASE ILLUSTRATION

To illustrate some of the ideas discussed in this chapter, we describe a case that presented in our clinic. When Sam, a 4-year-old African American boy, came to our clinic, he had a history of expulsions from three daycare centers and was in danger of being expelled from his current preschool due to his volatile behavior. Specifically, Sam was frequently aggressive with teachers and peers. For example, he often had tantrums that were so intense that his teachers would clear the classroom to ensure the safety of his classmates. Sam's parents were referred to the clinic by their pediatrician, who suggested rule-out diagnoses of ADHD, ODD, bipolar disorder, and even child-onset schizophrenia (because his tantrums appeared to mimic the meltdowns seen in children displaying psychotic behaviors).

Sam's parents, both college educated, were somewhat reluctant to seek psychological services, and this reluctance was evidenced by comments such as, "Sam is just a spirited child", and "Some of his teachers just didn't like him". As a result, the clinician initiated a frank discussion about their concerns and expectations and assured them that she would try to thoroughly explain each step in the assessment process. The parents were strongly encouraged to ask questions and raise concerns at any time. Sam's parents indicated that part of their reluctance was based on their concern that as an African American child, Sam would be subject to prejudice. In addition, they were concerned that he would be more quickly labeled as "stupid" and "bad" by a psychologist, as well as medicated unnecessarily or put in "slow kids' classes". Having this discussion with the parents allowed to clinician to develop a better understanding of the role the family's culture was playing in their reluctance to seek therapeutic services. The clinician addressed these concerns by asking the parents to recall times when they felt that they or their child had been subjected to this sort of cultural or racial bias. Sam's father reported that he experienced some learning difficulties in elementary school and was inappropriately placed in a classroom with emotionally handicapped children. This reportedly resulted in a battle between his parents and the school district. Consequently, this event clearly affected Sam's father's ability to trust schools and related professionals regarding his son's behavioral problems. Sam's parents were therefore caught in a "catch 22", that is, they wanted to get appropriate help for Sam, but they were convinced that the people who were offering help were going to hurt him by mislabeling him or placing him in incorrect classes. Through the use of empathic statements to validate their experiences and concerns, the clinician was able to indicate an awareness of and an appreciation for their dilemma. An explanation of the steps that would be taken to avoid bias while assessing Sam (i.e., careful interpretation of standardized forms, asking the parents about their thoughts of normative behavior in their culture, etc.) served to further reassure the parents that the clinician was sensitive to their family's cultural differences and would make every effort to accurately formulate the diagnosis and treatment plan for Sam.

Sam's formal assessment included parent and teacher standardized reports, clinical interviews with his parents and teachers, and observations of Sam in the classroom and the clinic. From these assessment techniques, psychotic and mood disorders (including schizophrenia and bipolar disorders) were ruled out. Specifically, Sam's behavior seemed clearly tied to inconsistent rewards and relatively few consequences for bad behavior. Therefore, Sam was given a diagnosis of ODD, and behavioral management techniques were used, based on the treatment manual *Parenting the Strong-Willed Child*,[6] an empirically supported treatment for children diagnosed with ODD.

Although the parent training principles were followed closely, the clinician used her dynamic sizing skills to make modifications to the standard treatment protocol to accommodate unique cultural characteristics of the family. One such characteristic was the involvement of the extended family in providing care for Sam. For example, Sam's grandmother often cared for him after school and for extended periods of time on weekends. Therefore, we made a summary sheet of each session with an abbreviated list of steps that the grandmother could use when taking care of Sam, in order to ensure that consistent behavioral goals and contingencies were in place. In addition, Sam was often surrounded by many family members and family friends who lavished him with presents and attention, regardless of his behavior. In order to make the behavioral contingencies effective, Sam's parents had to ask their relatives and friends to curb their present giving for the time being and simply give affection when Sam was using an acceptable range of appropriate behavior. This was a challenge for his parents because they thought that their friends and family would view this as an insult. Accordingly, time during several sessions was set aside to solve the problem about the most effective and least insulting way to communicate these behavior management goals to their loved ones. Fortunately, the clinician treating Sam's family knew when to appropriately individualize the treatment protocol to handle the unique situations of the family.

Another issue that presented an opportunity for culturally informed therapeutic intervention was that the parents were from a very high SES African American family, and they were apparently affected by the stereotypes about low SES African Americans that they held. This adversely affected their willingness to use effective parenting techniques. For example, prior to treatment, Sam would became very demanding when shopping with his parents and would generally have a very loud and dramatic tantrum if his parents refused to give in to his demands. His parents often responded by giving in to his demands (which is common in families caught in a coercive cycle with an oppositional child), thus reinforcing his behavior and guaranteeing future similar struggles. When instructed to ignore his disruptive store behavior in an effort to extinguish these tantrums, his parents were reluctant because, in their words, "We don't want to look like other African American parents who have children who scream in stores and who yell at and sometimes spank their children". Instead they chose to purchase him whatever he wanted to keep him quiet so that they would seem less, in their words, "ghetto" to other (primarily Caucasian) shoppers. To challenge Sam's parents' misconception that only African American children scream and throw fits in stores, the clinician asked them to complete a homework assignment that included observing parents and children in a toy store for an hour and recording the number of screaming Caucasian and African American children. Not surprisingly, Sam's parents reported no differences in numbers – children of all races and ethnicities were demanding and threw fits in toy stores. The clinician again used her dynamic sizing skills to understand that the family's culture was impacting their parenting skills. This knowledge allowed the clinician to individualize the treatment protocol to the unique situation of the family. Moreover, she took a scientifically minded approach and taught the family to test their hypothesis about screaming children. The clinician and Sam's parents also had a brief conversation about how their attempts to distance themselves from "ghetto" African American culture could adversely affect their ability to effectively care for their child. Consequently, they were more motivated to follow the parent training techniques in spite of their occasional discomfort with them.

Sam's parents became more confident in their parenting abilities and continued to follow the parenting techniques learned in therapy, including ignoring Sam's disruptive behaviors and establishing a point system to reward Sam's positive behaviors. Three months after beginning therapy and the implementation of behavioral management techniques, Sam no longer met criteria for ODD – just in time for him to begin kindergarten at a new school. At a follow-up (approximately three months into the new school year), Sam's parents reported that he had no behavior problems and that he was excelling academically. In addition, he was even recommended for an evaluation for the enriched education program. Furthermore, Sam's father indicated that he and his wife had enthusiastically shared the point system from the parent training therapy with parents of Sam's cousins and friends. In short, this resulted in the adoption of similar systems in many of these parents' households, as well as similar success stories.

CONCLUSIONS AND FUTURE DIRECTIONS

Although behavioral parent training is widely accepted as an effective treatment for children with externalizing problem behaviors, it is not equally effective or practical for all families. Modifications of the assessment and the diagnostic and treatment processes may be essential due to the differences that exist between families. Culturally competent clinicians possess knowledge of the differences that may exist between families from diverse backgrounds and the role these differences may play in behavioral parent training. Some of these differences have been highlighted in this chapter, such as culture, race or ethnicity, SES/resource availability, and family structure. Further, this chapter is certainly not an exhaustive list of all the possible variables that may influence the efficacy of behavioral parent training among diverse families. Overall, more research is clearly needed on these factors as well as other variables that may moderate and mediate treatment effects.

The lens through which behavior is viewed is influenced heavily by cultural norms.[13] Values and beliefs about parenting that are specific to certain cultures will impact the way children's behavior is viewed and reported. In addition, treatment occurs within the larger context of family groups and culture, and clinicians need to be aware of and sensitive to cultural differences if they want success in changing dysfunctional parenting behavior or child misbehavior. A lack of competence or sensitivity to cultural differences may have deleterious effects on aspects of the treatment process, such as completion of homework assignments, consistent use of empirically supported parenting techniques, and therapeutic alliance. Moreover, cultural competence and culture-specific expertise[7] allow the clinician to view the client in a nonjudgmental manner, thereby building rapport and enhancing the therapeutic alliance. In fact, if parent training is viewed by the parents as a method of shaping the child's behavior into conformity with the mainstream beliefs about parenting, the treatment will likely be unsuccessful.[11] Rather, this treatment should be presented as a way for parents to manage their child's behavior in an effective manner that is consistent with their values and beliefs.

However, it is important to remember that substantial differences exist *within* each culture. In fact, differences between families of the same race, ethnicity, SES, or family structure may be greater than differences between groups. Clinicians should never assume that a family that identifies with a given cultural group, possesses an atypical family structure, or belongs to a certain SES will behave a certain way. Scientifically minded clinicians develop and test cultural hypotheses in order to determine if generalizations can be made.[7]

Most empirical studies of behavioral parent training have used largely Caucasian samples. When minorities are included in studies, the roles of ethnicity and culture are rarely viewed as specific contextual variables that help explain behavior.[50] Research studies of behavioral parent training have begun to include culturally diverse samples; however, the next step is to examine culture as a central explanatory variable. Future studies should compare the effectiveness of behavioral parent training with minority cultures compared with majority cultures. If differences are found between groups, culture should be examined as a potential explanatory variable. Researchers also need to empirically examine how well standard behavioral parent training techniques are accepted in different cultures.

The few studies that have examined differences in treatment outcome have found no differences between culturally diverse groups.[26,27] However, given the differences in parenting values that exist between different cultures, it is likely that groups will respond differently to behavioral parent training techniques that were developed using predominantly Caucasian samples. Although the basic components of behavioral parent training will likely be effective with most families, tailoring of the general technique to address a particular family's variables (e.g., SES, race, ethnicity, family structure) will likely maximize its efficacy and appeal to clients. Clinicians who possess culture-specific expertise and dynamic sizing skills know when it is appropriate to apply knowledge of a particular family's culture to the child's behavior and modify the standard treatment protocol.[7]

When treating families, clinicians will be more successful if they consider cultural, socioeconomic, and structural variables of the family. If a clinician has a narrow set of criteria for defining a functional family, few families may actually meet those criteria, and treatment success is less likely. Parent training will also be more successful if clinicians consider factors of the family and the system that shape parenting behavior and child behavior. In conclusion, clinicians and researchers who are competent in attending to the broader context of parenting will be maximally effective.

CHAPTER 7

The Assessment, Diagnosis, and Treatment of Psychiatric Disorders in Individuals with a Dual Diagnosis: the Co-occurrence of Developmental Disorders and Psychiatric Disorders

Robert C Schlauch, Kathryn H Gordon, and Norman B Schmidt

Approximately two decades ago, Reiss et al.[1] noted that "Mentally retarded people who are also emotionally disturbed may constitute one of the most underserved populations in the United States" (p. 361). This assertion was based on a growing recognition that individuals with mental retardation (MR) were vulnerable to a wide range of mental health problems, which often are not properly identified or responded to with appropriate services.[2] Reiss et al.[1] delineated some of the potential mechanisms that may serve to increase risk for mental health problems in individuals with MR, as well as some conceptual, administrative, and attitudinal reasons that may limit mental health service utilization in this population. They concluded that individuals with MR potentially suffer from two related outcomes owing to low intelligence: (i) the increased risk for emotional disturbance, and (ii) the decreased opportunity for adequate treatment.[1]

Since Reiss et al.'s[1] review, studies have more definitively documented the first risk. That is, individuals with MR indeed show a high prevalence of emotional and behavioral problems. However, relatively little empirical study has been devoted to the second issue – that is, increasing opportunities for people with MR to receive adequate mental health services. Empirical studies examining such issues in pervasive developmental disorders (PDDs) such as autism and Asperger's disorder are even more scarce. However, there is reason to believe that many of the issues that arise for those with MR and comorbid psychiatric diagnoses are similar to those for other PDDs.

Research has often referred to this population as having a dual diagnosis to indicate the co-occurrence of MR as well as a psychiatric disturbance. For the purposes of this chapter, dual diagnosis will also be used to indicate those with the co-occurrence of MR or any PDD and a psychiatric disturbance. Thus, the aim of this chapter is to review the current literature on the assessment, diagnosis, and treatment of those with a dual diagnosis, as well as to provide case examples illustrating some of the issues that may arise.

GENERAL BACKGROUND INFORMATION

As cited in the DSM-IV, public law 95-602 (1978) defined a developmental disability as "a disability attributable to a mental or physical impairment, manifested before the age of 22, likely to continue indefinitely, resulting in substantial limitation in three or more specific areas of functioning, and requiring specific and lifelong or extended care . . ." (p. 45).[3] Included under the category of developmental disabilities are both MR and PDDs. The *Diagnostic and Statistical Manual of Mental Disorders*, fourth edition (DSM-IV-TR) defines MR as "significantly subaverage general intellectual functioning that is accompanied by significant limitations in adaptive functioning in at least two of the following skill areas: communication, self-care, home living, social skills, self-direction, functional academic skills, work, leisure, health, and safety" (p. 41).[4] PDDs are characterized "by severe and pervasive impairment in several areas of development; reciprocal social interaction skills, communication skills, or the presence of stereotypic behavior, interests, and activities".[4] Such disorders include autistic disorder, Asperger's disorder, Rett's disorder, childhood disintegrative disorder, and PDD not otherwise specified. The most common of these are autistic and Asperger's disorders.

Research has demonstrated that those with MR or a PDD are at a greater risk for the development of psychological problems than the general public.[5-9] A number of studies have directly compared the rates of psychopathology for people with and without MR. One of the earliest studies was conducted on the Isle of Wight in the United Kingdom.[10] This research was based on a survey of the entire population of children aged 9–11 years. A two-step methodology was used. In step 1, screening questionnaires were completed by teachers and parents. In step 2, interviews and other data were collected from both parents and teachers on the child. Approximately 30% of children diagnosed as having MR were diagnosed with an additional comorbid disorder based on parent interviews, and 42% based on teacher ratings. These results indicate a five to seven times greater risk for developing psychiatric diagnoses in children with MR than for children without MR.

Furthermore, researchers have found that perhaps as many as a third or more of all people with MR have a significant behavioral, mental, or personality disorder requiring mental health services.[6] For example, Goldberg et al.[7] reported that in 384 Canadians with MR, 257 (67%) meet criteria for at least one comorbid psychiatric disorder, which is more than twice that seen in the general public (in which 26.2% suffer from a diagnosable psychiatric disorder in a given year).[11] Specifically, 88 (23%) had adjustment disorders, 43 (11%) impulse control disorders, 25 (6.5%) depressive disorders, 19 (5%) psychotic disorders, and 14 (4%) had anxiety disorders. Given a prevalence rate of MR of about 12% of the total population – or about three to six million people in the United States – there may be as many as one to two million Americans who have both MR and a mental health disorder.[2]

Research on prevalence rates of comorbid psychiatric diagnoses in other PDDs, such as Asperger's disorder, is fairly limited. Despite the limited research, studies have consistently demonstrated that those with a PDD are at greater risk for the development of comorbid psychiatric disorders.[8,9,12] For example, Ghaziuddin and colleagues[9] found that in a sample of 35 patients diagnosed with Asperger's disorder, 23 (65%) presented with symptoms of an additional psychiatric disorder at the time of initial evaluation or during the two-year follow-up. Thus, those with other PDDs may also be at increased risk for developing mental health problems.

Overall, studies on rates of dual diagnosis (i.e., diagnosis of a developmental disability and at least one other comorbid psychiatric disorder) have indicated a wide variation in reported rates, ranging from under 15% to over 35%. A number of factors have been suggested as possible explanations for this variation.[6,13] These factors include differences in sampling techniques,[14] differences in classification systems,[13] and differences in the comprehensiveness of rating instruments.[15] Reiss[15] suggested that low prevalence estimates of such dual diagnoses were obtained in studies that relied on surveys of case files, whereas high prevalence estimates of dual diagnosis were obtained in studies that used professional interviewers. Consistent with this suggestion, Reiss[15] found that for every individual who has a mental health disorder recorded in his or her case file, there are an estimated two to three who have an undiagnosed mental health disorder. At least three factors may account for this apparent underdiagnosis of mental health disorders in people with MR and PDDs. First, the vulnerability of people with MR and PDDs to psychopathology was not fully recognized prior to the mid-1980s. Consequently, there were many people with mental health disorders who were not referred for a psychiatric evaluation. In such cases, the mental health disorder would be detected in a research study in which the subjects were interviewed but perhaps not in a research survey of historical case files. Second, there has been a shortage of trained psychiatrists interested in working with people with MR and PDDs. There were many past instances in which a psychiatric diagnosis was not made simply because a psychiatrist was not available to evaluate the individual. In such cases, psychopathology might be detected in a research study in which the subjects were interviewed by psychiatrists or psychologists but not in a research survey of historical case files. Finally, the phenomenon of *diagnostic overshadowing*[16] suggests a general tendency to underdiagnose mental health disorders in persons with MR. In diagnostic overshadowing, professionals may presume that the behavioral problems of people with MR are a consequence of the MR rather than evidence of a separate mental illness. Because of diagnostic overshadowing, there could be many people with MR or a PDD who had psychiatric and behavioral disorders that were not diagnosed separately from that condition.

In addition, another issue that complicates the identification of comorbid diagnoses in those with MR and PDDs is linguistic barriers. As mentioned earlier, individuals with MR and PDDs often have impairments in social and communication skills, and thus may have difficulty expressing themselves. Moss[17] points out that linguistic barriers complicate efforts to obtain accurate diagnoses, mainly because of an over-reliance on third-party reports and observations for diagnostic information, an issue that clinicians need to be aware of when conducting assessments and formulating diagnoses. However, this does not mean that assessing, diagnosing, and treating those with a dual diagnosis is an impossible task. It merely suggests that one needs to be very mindful of possible issues that may arise. Thus, this chapter will focus on issues one should consider when working with this unique and diverse population. We will discuss assessment, diagnosis, and treatment of comorbid diagnoses (e.g., anxiety, depression) based on our experience with treating such a population, followed by a section reviewing some of the current literature in these areas. Finally, we will present a comprehensive case example that will tie together many of these issues and how they may play out in a case.

CLINICAL OBSERVATIONS
Assessment

Nisbett and Ross[18] point out that the human ability to draw inferences is flawed and biased, as a result of prior experiences and beliefs influencing opinions. Furthermore, they point out that many times people rely on human intuition, and that human intuition is also flawed. But what does this all mean for mental health practitioners? For one, practitioners need to be aware of such biases as they will be the ones making diagnoses and recommendations for treatments. It also warns that clients themselves can be biased in reporting symptoms. Because of this fact, clinicians must use assessment procedures that are both subjective and objective. Using objective measures will help reduce biases and flaws in human decision making. It is important to note that this practice will not eliminate all biases, and in fact other biases in judgment such as what assessment tools should be used, how to interpret their results, and how to apply assessment results may be present.

Assessments can be used for forming diagnoses, as well as formulating and evaluating treatments. Treatment utility of assessment has been defined as the "degree to which assessment is shown to contribute to beneficial treatment outcome."[19] The treatment application of assessment can occur in many different ways, including the identification of functional or causal relationships, the assessment of whether treatment is failing or working, the definition of treatment outcomes, and the identification of targeted behaviors. Diagnostic clinical examinations should contain three basic components: (i) a detailed history; (ii) a direct interview; and (iii) diagnostic formulation based on information obtained (i.e., convergence of evidence from information obtained from assessment, discussed more in the next section, Diagnosis).[20] Standard practice in any clinic with regard to assessment should be a multi-method, multi-informant approach. Multi-method, multi-informant assessment refers to the use of many types of assessment method (i.e., self-report measures, standardized tests, clinical interview) and having more than one person reporting on such information. The advantage of using multiple methods of assessment is that it minimizes error associated with any one method and evaluates the convergence across the different measures, whereas having multiple informants helps minimize the biases of any one single informant, provides information in various situations (e.g., home and work), and assists with the developmental limitations that are associated with those with a dual diagnosis. Such an approach appears to be particularly relevant in being able to assess clients with a dual diagnosis, given the particular barriers that may come up with clients who have limited verbal or intellectual abilities.

Currently, there are various methods of assessment that a clinician can use while gathering information. However, one must be realistic in acknowledging that some methods may not be available to the clinician, as well as recognizing that some assessment procedures may be very time consuming. Further, it is important that clinicians know when it is appropriate to use certain assessment techniques and when not to. Sue[21] points out in his article on cultural competency in psychotherapy and counseling that clinicians need to know when it is appropriate to generalize and be inclusive, verses when to individualize and be exclusive. By understanding this principle, which is referred to as dynamic sizing, clinicians will be able to avoid over generalizing based on their knowledge of that population (i.e., stereotyping) and appreciate individual differences. Thus, clinicians should not allow stereotypes of a specific population to influence what measures and assessment methods to use, but rather they should adapt to the needs of the client. This assessment process will vary from client to client, but first and foremost there should always be a clinical interview with the client. Szymanski and colleagues[20] point out that "a direct interview with the referred is essential. Lack of verbal language is a reason for a longer, not shorter, interview which may also include observing the person in work and living conditions" (p. 7). For those who are higher functioning and have reasonable verbal skills, such an interview will follow typical assessment procedures with minor modifications based on developmental levels. With the consent of the client, it may be beneficial to have a third party (i.e., friend or family member) present to add information that the client may have difficulty expressing. However, with those who are lower functioning and have poor communication skills, informants may become an absolute necessity during such a process.

Szymanski et al.[20] noted that observations in various settings may be important. As will be discussed in the diagnostic considerations section, those who are lower functioning will most likely display more behavior problems and have more somatic complaints rather than the traditional symptoms presented in the DSM-IV. As such, behavioral observations, particularly functional assessments, become essential. Functional assessment is a way of measuring and analyzing behaviors as they occur in the client's daily environments. Such a process involves the identification of behavioral antecedents, actual behaviors, and consequences of such behaviors. Problematic behaviors may be identified using functional assessment techniques that indicate psychopathology. For example, a person with MR or a PDD who has difficulty with verbal communication may exhibit behavior problems to avoid situations that elicit fear and anxiety. Functional assessments may be able to identify such behaviors by understanding the situational context in which the behaviors occur and what the resulting consequences are of such behaviors. Such a process allows clinicians to form and test hypotheses rather than draw conclusions prematurely solely based on this population's unique differences, a principle referred to as scientific mindedness.[21] Further, application of skills of scientific mindedness may also prevent issues of diagnostic overshadowing, in that clinicians will no longer assume that behavioral problems of people with MR or PDD are a consequence of the MR or PDD.

Self-report measures may also provide valuable information to diagnose a condition and plan a treatment for individuals with a dual diagnosis. It is recommended that standardized measures be used whenever possible in order to help eliminate biases related to clinical intuition and subjectivity. Again, it is important that clinicians do not allow their knowledge of the population they are assessing to fully determine the types of assessment to use or influence the way such measures are interpreted (i.e., dynamic sizing). When the client has reasonable verbal skills and is higher functioning, such self-report measures may provide accurate information. However, this may not always be the case. For example, the case example presented later demonstrates that although the client with Asperger's disorder (being treated for major depression and generalized anxiety disorder) had above average intellectual ability, he had difficulty understanding the emotional content of the questions in a self-report measure. He was better able to relate to the behavioral symptoms during a clinical interview. Additional measures that clinicians may want to consider administering are standardized symptom checklists that are completed by third parties familiar with the client. However, such measures have a variety of limitations and should never be the sole source for assessing diagnostic symptoms (issues that will be discussed later).

Diagnosis

Two questions should be kept in mind when considering diagnostic criteria:[20]

- To what extent is it possible to establish psychiatric diagnosis, according to standard diagnostic classification, for people who have a dual diagnosis?
- What modifications of diagnostic criteria might be needed to diagnose mental disorders in people with MR?

There is now a general consensus that those with MR or PDDs can be diagnosed with comorbid psychiatric disorders, particularly when such individuals are higher functioning and have reasonable communicative skills.[2] However, diagnostic presentation may not be the same for individuals with MR or PDDs due to their lower intellectual functioning and/or poor communication skills. One useful approach clinicians can take with regards to issues of diagnostic criteria in such a population is referring to literature on developmental psychopathology.

Developmental psychopathology has been defined as the study of clinical dysfunction over the course of development and in the context of maturational and developmental processes.[22] It considers not only cognitive development, but also affective and physiological development. Because MR and PDDs are characterized by impairment in several areas of development, such as communication skills, reciprocal social interaction skills, and MR is characterized by impairments in general intellectual functioning, using a developmental psychopathology framework may prove to be very useful. Understanding the developmental level of a patient will most likely be the key to whether an additional diagnosis is warranted. Not surprisingly, the DSM-IV criteria on most disorders were developed based on individuals without significant developmental delays, and as such, some criteria may not apply to individuals with MR and PDDs. As the developmental psychopathology literature points out, children with disorders are not just "little adult" equivalents.[23] The same can be said for those with MR and PDDs. That is, symptoms of psychopathology may vary as a function of the developmental level of an individual, for which many diagnostic criteria currently do not account.

For those who are higher functioning and have adequate verbal skills, current DSM-IV diagnostic criteria will most likely be appropriate in identifying individuals with comorbid diagnoses. However, those who are lower functioning and/or have poor communication skills may display more behavioral problems and somatic complaints. For example, one criterion for major depressive disorder (MDD) is the presence of a depressed mood most of the day, as indicated by either subjective reports or observations made by others. One example of the way this symptom may manifest in an individual with MR is if his or her caregiver's descriptions change from the client being happy and smiling or laughing or having a sense of humor to a distinct absence of these characteristics. Other possibilities are tearfulness, an increase in somatic complaints (such as difficulty sleeping or change in appetite), and irritability. Further, sleep difficulties may not mimic pure insomnia or hypersomnia, but rather behavioral disturbances in the evening (e.g., resistance to go to bed on time). Although individuals with MR or PDDs may have difficulty verbalizing such feelings and emotions, other symptoms may be present that indicate such problems. Thus, a good rule of thumb when considering diagnostic criteria is to consider the presence, persistence, pervasiveness, and impairment of such symptoms in the context of developmental processes. That is, compared with others with MR or PDDs, are these behaviors/symptoms "abnormal?"

Treatment

Therapists working with this population may be prone to burnout and fatigue, because the therapeutic process can be quite challenging with individuals with MR or PDDs. Thus, it is essential that therapists are mindful of the client's limitations when developing goals for treatment. For many clients, the goal of therapy is full remission of the symptoms of their mental disorder. Clearly this is not possible, or at least highly unlikely, when one of their mental disorders is MR or a PDD. When working with clients with dual diagnosis, it is useful to establish what their best possible functioning would look like, and use that as a goal of treatment. One way to establish this is to ask the client (or other informants) to pinpoint the "best time" in the client's life, and how they were feeling and functioning at that time. For example, the treatment goal for a client who presented with MR and depression symptoms was to improve his functioning such that he could resume daily activities such as chores, helping his family with dinner, and participating in church activities.

Realistic expectations are important for both the therapist and the client, because striving for unattainable goals could result in both parties feeling frustrated, pessimistic, and ineffective. It is therefore particularly important to continually assess progress of any type, so that that the client and therapist can see where functioning has improved and determine whether the treatment approach being used is effective. It is worth noting that therapists may experience frustration with clients who make slower progress at times, and that this is a natural response, but action should be taken to prevent this from negatively impacting therapy. One way to do this is for therapists to take the client's perspective when they begin feeling frustrated. For example, a therapist was becoming frustrated with her adolescent client's difficulty remembering information from session to session. The client must have sensed this, and said, "I am doing the best I can do. I wish I could remember everything you said." The therapist immediately returned to a compassionate stance, and was humbled by the comment. When becoming frustrated or burned out with slow progress in therapy, falling back on empathy can improve the therapeutic relationship. It is important that a clinician place the client's behavior in the proper context. The therapist must be aware of times when it is and is not appropriate to apply their knowledge of the client's intellectual and/ or social limitations to their particular client's behavior. In this case, a therapist must recognize that the client may experience extreme difficulty due to their developmental disability (i.e., dynamic sizing).

Once realistic treatment goals have been established, it is recommended that therapy include a substantial behavioral component in conjunction with cognitive therapy. Because clients with MR or PDDs may have difficulty with traditional cognitive therapy concepts, they may benefit from a treatment plan that includes pure behavioral techniques (e.g., behavioral activation, behavioral modification systems). It is important to note that many behavioral techniques alone have been empirical supported as a primary treatment for psychiatric disorders (e.g., exposure, behavioral activation). This component may be particularly important when cognitive modes are less effective.

The Cognitive Behavioral Analysis System of Psychotherapy (CBASP)[24] may be a particularly useful therapeutic technique with this population. CBASP focuses on brief interpersonal situations (e.g., 15–30 minutes), and asks the client to describe the situation in behavioral terms (e.g., "How would a fly on the wall describe the situation?"). CBASP devotes relatively less attention to emotional and cognitive aspects, and involves teaching the client to focus on what their desired outcome in a situation is, and what behaviors will help them to attain their desired outcome. The narrow focus and concrete nature of this technique may appeal to clients with PDDs who have adequate verbal abilities.

Individuals with MR and PDDs are often more prone to social skills deficits and may struggle with appropriate eye contact, reciprocal conversation, and personal space issues. CBASP is a well-suited framework for these issues, where the therapist and client can work together to determine what behaviors were helpful or hurtful to the client's chances of achieving their goals in interpersonal situations. In addition to using CBASP to address social skills issues, it may be helpful for the therapist to provide feedback to the client about appropriate interactions in session. For example, one of our therapists said to the client, "I like how you're making eye contact with me now. It shows me that you're listening."

The involvement of family members and loved ones in treatment may be particularly beneficial in working with clients with MR and PDDs. Providing psychoeducation for the people who interact with the client about their psychological conditions and treatment plan could serve to generalize skills learned in therapy to other settings. The therapist can act as an advocate for their client, collaborating with people in their workplace and/or home to develop ways to make the working and home environment optimal for the client's functioning.

Finally, clients may benefit from taking psychiatric medications that have empirical support for efficacy in individuals without MR or PDDs. Psychotic, anxious, and depressive symptoms, in addition to certain behavioral problems (e.g., impulse control), may be ameliorated with the use of psychotropic medications. Here again, it is important that the effects of medication – both therapeutic and potential negative side effects – be monitored carefully. Information derived from behavioral observations and multiple informants, when available, is the best way to provide information about effectiveness. To date, no large-scale randomized clinical trials have been conducted with medications in developmentally disabled individuals with comorbid mental health problems. Sevin et al.[25] have published a theoretical paper outlining the studies that need to be conducted to evaluate the potential benefits of pharmacological treatments in developmentally disabled individuals, including specific techniques for determining the potential benefits of using pharmacological interventions in conjunction with psychosocial interventions. They provide a springboard for future theory-driven studies of the effectiveness of medication in this population.

THE CURRENT STATE OF THE LITERATURE
Assessment

Reid[26] suggests that commonly used assessment procedures should be a starting point for assessment regardless of any special issues; however, these procedures then need to be modified to accommodate the client. It is important for the clinician not to assume that, because of the intellectual/social limitations of their clients, commonly used assessment procedures cannot be used. Rather, they should use such knowledge to modify such techniques to meet that client's needs (i.e., dynamic sizing). In particular, when assessing individuals with MR and PDDs, the consensus is that assessment should include several components. These components include a review of client records, interviews, observations, and rating scales.[27-29] Although numerous measures have been developed to aid in the diagnosis of psychiatric disorders in populations with MR, little empirical research has been conducted on the clinical utility of such measures. The five more common and well-researched measures include: the Psychopathology Interview for Mentally Retarded Adults (PIMRA),[30] the Diagnostic Assessment for Severely Handicapped (DASH-II),[31] the Reiss Screen for Maladaptive Behavior (RSMB),[32] the Psychiatric Assessment Schedule for Adults with Developmental Disabilities Checklist (PAS-ADD Checklist),[33] and the Aberrant Behavior Checklist (ABC).[34] Reviews of these instruments have come to the conclusion that many of these measures' psychometric properties have not been tested thoroughly and tend to have a limited range of content.[27,35] Specifically, Aman[27] concluded that for many of the available measures (i) the sensitivity and specificity are largely unknown, (ii) the diagnostic accuracy is largely unknown, and (iii) standardization of such measures is generally inadequate, as they are developed and tested on relatively small populations. These findings indicate that although these measures were developed with this population in mind, many limitations to such measures have not been well researched, and as such, one must be cautious of using such measures. Further, many of these measures were developed for those with MR, and have not been tested on those with other PDDs.

It has been suggested that functional assessment techniques, including the use of behavioral descriptive instruments, are essential in the diagnosis of comorbid psychiatric disorders in clients with MR.[29,36] Such an assessment technique may prove to be very important given the higher rates of behavioral problems in this population, and the uncertainty of how psychopathology is represented in such a population. Further, observations of routine behaviors has recently become of interest to researchers. For example, Green and Reid[37] attempted to operationalize happiness/unhappiness in individuals based on the frequency of behaviors indicative of such affective states (smiling, laughing, crying, frowning, etc.). These behaviors were observed in the context of identified activities and objects known to be enjoyable to the client. The results of their study indicated that observing such behaviors was a valid means of measuring happiness in individuals with MR. Importantly, these findings have been replicated.[38,39] As a result, some researchers have begun to use such a measure of happiness to monitor changes in mood during the implementation of behavioral treatments.[40,41] Although these studies did not use such measures specifically to aid in diagnosis, they demonstrated that such measures are valid and can be used to assess the progress of treatment in such populations. Also, it suggests that certain simple behaviors (such as frequency of smiling) may also be a means of assessing symptomatology of psychiatric disorders in those with MR or PDDs by observing how such behaviors may change over time.

Diagnosis

One reason that there is an underdiagnosis of psychiatric disorders in individuals with MR and PDDs may be due to the inadequacy of the current diagnostic system for use with this population.[29] The most common diagnostic system used today is the DSM.[4] The DSM relies on subjective report for assessment of much of the symptomatology. Modifications may be needed because individuals with MR or PDDs often have difficulty with verbal communication.

A review of the literature revealed little empirical research on symptom presentations and diagnostic considerations for those with MR and PDDs. Research has suggested that those who are higher functioning and who have adequate verbal skills tend to have symptom presentations similar to the general population. For example, in one study generalized anxiety disorder (GAD) in mildly developmentally delayed people largely paralleled that of nondelayed people, except for brooding, somatic complaints, and sleep disorders, all of which were more common in those with MR.[42] However, research on symptom presentation for those with lower intellectual abilities and poorer communication skills is severely lacking. Aman[27] reviewed available assessment instruments, and noted that the expression of psychopathology may change in ways not yet understood in populations with MR and PDD, particularly in those who are lower functioning, and that even among those in the mild range of intellectual disability, clinical presentation will vary.

One way in which clinical presentation of psychiatric disorders may be different is that those with MR and PDDs may display more behavioral problems versus traditional symptoms of psychopathology (i.e., DSM criteria). Consistent with this, research has found that those with MR exhibit high rates of behavior problems. For example, Deb et al.[43] found that out of 100 10–64-year-olds diagnosed with MR, 60% had at least one behavior disorder, with such behaviors including aggression, self-injurious behaviors, objectionable habits, night-time disturbances and destructiveness. However, little research has been conducted in an attempt to link such behaviors to symptoms of psychiatric disorders. Thus, the current DSM-IV-TR may not be representative for those with MR or PDDs, and one should be mindful of such limitations.

Treatment

Benson[44] recently reviewed psychological interventions that have been used with clients who are dually diagnosed with intellectual disabilities and psychiatric disorders. The review concluded that there are sparse data on the efficacy of psychological interventions for psychiatric disorders in individuals with intellectual disabilities. Benson[44] identified some key obstacles to this line of research. First, clinical trials in this population would require longer spans of times than typical clinical trials, because it usually takes a longer period of time to observe changes in symptoms. Longer trials would require more time, money, and resources. Second, there could be special ethical issues that arise, such as challenges in obtaining informed consent and withholding treatment to form a control group. Third, this group of individuals is diverse in presentation. Thus, balancing the need for a homogeneous sample in order to establish efficacy with the need for the intervention to generalize to real-world circumstances (which is important for establishing effectiveness)[45] is particularly challenging with this group of individuals. Finally, as mentioned in the section on diagnosis, disorder presentation may differ in individuals with intellectual disabilities, and thus a modified classification system may be needed with this population. As a result of these challenges, there are limited data on patients with intellectual disabilities, and often the studies that do exist have flaws in their design that make their findings difficult to rely upon.

Benson[44] highlighted two recent reviews of the treatment of individuals with dual diagnosis. The first, by Prout and Nowak-Drabik,[46] reviewed 92 studies on therapeutic intervention conducted between 1968 and 1998. The vast majority of these studies were case studies or single case designs, and many studies did not have specific details about the intervention and client characteristics. In addition, standardized measures were often not included in the studies. These limitations must be considered when weighing the impact of their conclusions. Prout and Nowak-Drabik[46] used meta-analytic procedures on the nine studies that provided enough information for computation of effect size. These nine studies utilized a variety of psychological interventions (e.g., skills training, cognitive-behavioral, humanistic) to address various psychiatric problems. Results indicated a mean effect size of 1.0 standard deviation improvement in post-treatment symptoms. Again, this finding should be considered with caution in light of the aforementioned limitations of the studies that were reviewed.

Second, Beail[47] reviewed the literature that had been published since 1996, and focused on studies about the effectiveness of either psychodynamic or cognitive-behavioral intervention with individuals with intellectual disabilities. One limitation of this review is that Beail did not use statistical measures, but rather a descriptive analysis of the studies. Beail concluded that group designs often lacked sufficient power to detect group differences, and that groups were often not homogeneous. The main contribution of this paper was the conclusion that there continues to be slow progress in how to treat individuals with intellectual disabilities, and the research is drastically lagging behind other lines of treatment research. Thus, the review makes the need for well-designed research in this population even more apparent.

Benson's[44] review highlighted five case studies of individuals with intellectual disabilities (one client had Down's syndrome and the other four clients had "moderate to severe intellectual disabilities") and various mental health issues (dog phobia, selective mutism, borderline personality disorder, bereavement, and aggressive/self-harm behaviors). All five clients experienced significant improvement in their functioning. Clearly, there are important limitations to consider when gleaning information from case studies. Most importantly, it is much more likely that successful cases will be published in journals, and thus therapists cannot be certain that these interventions will generalize to most cases.

However, because of limited data in this area, case studies can provide ideas for what has been effective with some patients with intellectual disabilities, and may serve to form hypotheses to be tested in larger samples.

Across these cases, the findings are consistent with earlier assertions that empirically supported treatments, with some adaptations, may be effective in clients with intellectual disabilities, but the emphasis on more behavioral aspects of the techniques may be particularly important with this population. The five case studies yielded support for behavioral treatments that utilize functional analysis to decrease skills deficits and maladaptive behavior. In each of the five cases, target behaviors were identified, the functions of these behaviors were analyzed, and treatment techniques that were designed to target the behaviors successfully improved functioning.

For example, one case study describes a woman with moderate to severe intellectual disability who began exhibiting significant behavior problems after the loss of her father. The mental health professionals assessed the function of this behavior, and identified her problematic behavior as a way in which she was trying to cope with grief in the absence of appropriate coping skills. Twelve sessions of psychoeducation and processing of her grief feelings resulted in substantial behavioral improvement.[48] Another case study describes the treatment of an adolescent boy with a dog phobia. The individual was successfully treated using graded exposure to dogs, relaxation training, and vicarious modeling.[49] In addition, the inclusion of a family member in his treatment (his mother modeled nonphobic behavior with the dogs) seemed to have been effective in reducing his dog phobia symptoms.

Social skills deficits and poor interpersonal functioning are viewed as risk factors for developing mental disorders, in general,[50] and social skills deficits are, by definition, present in individuals diagnosed with PDDs. Among individuals with Asperger's disorder, those with more severe social disabilities are more prone to depression symptoms.[51] Early intervention with the focus of building social support networks and social skills may serve to buffer these individuals from the onset of depression as well as anxiety symptoms. One technique that has been used to enhance the ability to appropriately navigate social situations is Social Stories for children, which is similar to CBASP for adults and involves creating a short story that describes a situation and includes appropriate actions and expressions. Other common practices with children who have PDDs include arranging play dates, and increasing peer group tolerance.[52]

Currently, no treatments are well established for the treatment of social disabilities, but contingency management has received some empirical support. Contingency management attempts to change behavior by altering its consequences though behavioral principles such as shaping, positive reinforcement, and extinction.[53,54] Contingency management has been effectively used to increase social behaviors (e.g., good eye contact), and decrease negative social behaviors (e.g., standing too close to others). There are few empirical studies on treating depression and anxiety symptoms in individuals with PDDs, with a particular paucity of studies in the area of interventions for adults with autism spectrum disorders. Currently, it is recommended that empirically supported treatments be used with this population, and the adaptations mentioned above be considered, as there is some evidence that this is effective.[55]

COMPREHENSIVE CASE ILLUSTRATION

Patrick, a 37-year-old man diagnosed with Asperger's disorder, presented at an outpatient clinic because he had been experiencing depression and anxiety symptoms. Patrick had above average intelligence, as evidenced by scoring in the gifted range of intellectual abilities when he was tested as a child, and also by the fact that he had earned a master's degree in history. Impairments were observed in his ability to engage in reciprocal social interactions (e.g., infrequent eye contact, one-sided conversations, demonstrated stereotypic interests). He described that he was having difficulties transitioning into a new job, and that this led to sadness, sleep difficulty, increased perseverative thoughts, rapid heartbeat, and muscle tension. Patrick explained that he had had bouts of anxiety and depression since he was a child, and that he was hoping that therapy could help him to feel better. At screening, he explained that the anxiety and depression symptoms "exacerbated" his Asperger's disorder characteristics (e.g., difficulty reading nonverbal cues, becoming overwhelmed by stimuli) such that he felt social situations became increasingly difficult for him to navigate. Given the variability of the levels of functioning among this population, it is important to note that Patrick may be more representative of higher functioning clients. Thus, the current case presentation may not apply to individuals who are lower functioning.

Patrick completed self-report paper-and-pencil measures that tapped anxiety and depression symptoms (e.g., Beck Depression Inventory, Beck Anxiety Inventory). Despite having reported clinically significant anxiety and depression symptoms on his application, he scored in the mild range of symptoms on both measures. However, when followed up with a structured interview, Patrick met full criteria for MDD and GAD. When Patrick was asked about the discrepancy between the self-report measures and the interview information, he reported that he had some difficulty processing the emotional content of the questionnaires, whereas the interview was able to focus on more behavioral descriptions of symptoms (e.g., hours of sleep at night, change in eating patterns, muscle tension). It was determined that CBASP would be the best way to treat his symptoms, as many of his stressors were interpersonal in nature.

Therapy focused on Patrick's relationship difficulties, because his interpersonal struggles appeared to be the source of much of his distress. For example, Patrick frequently expected people to put more effort into helping and understanding him than they actually did. As a result, Patrick tended to send e-mails or make telephone calls criticizing people for their behavior. This behavior resulted in some of his co-workers telling him not to call or e-mail them again, or to restrict his contact to once a week.

Patrick completed weekly homework assignments (Coping Survey Questionnaires [CSQs], which ask for detailed descriptions including thoughts and behaviors of a brief interpersonal interaction; see McCullough[24]) and in-session exercises that taught him how to conceptualize situations in a CSQ format, such that Patrick could identify his desired outcome, and determine which thoughts and behaviors would increase his chances of achieving his desired outcome. Patrick struggled with completing the CSQs at first. He particularly had trouble staying focused on a specific situation. He often had difficulty taking the perspective of others, and appeared to lack insight into why his behavior seemed to lead to undesired reactions from others.

For example, Patrick was having difficulty understanding his responsibilities at work. As a result, he often spent evenings ruminating about possible mistakes he had made, and felt overwhelmed when he did not know how to complete a task. The therapist suggested that he invite his vocational coach to come into a therapy session, so that she could facilitate communication between them, and help in problem solving about occupational issues. At the session before the meeting, Patrick completed a prospective CSQ. Below is a transcript of the session.

Patrick (P): I have been having a lot of trouble at work. My vocational coach *should* be talking to my boss about my needs, but she isn't.

Therapist (T): It sounds like you're pretty frustrated. Have you tried talking to her about your concerns?

P: Well, I have tried a few times, but I end up getting nervous and frustrated, and it just seems to go nowhere.

T: You suggested that we invite your job coach to come in for a session, so that I could assist in problem solving.

P: Maybe she'll listen to you.

T: As we have discussed before, I want to help you to learn how to advocate for yourself. That way, when therapy ends, you will be skilled at asking for and getting what you need.

P: I am worried that I'll get overwhelmed and withdraw from the conversation like in the past.

T: I can understand why you would feel nervous. Why don't we try planning for the meeting by using the CSQ format that we have been using in therapy?

P: Okay, plans always make me to feel more comfortable.

T: What is your desired outcome for the meeting?

P: I want my job to be less stressful.

T: Okay, remember, for these exercises, it is important to pick a specific desired outcome for a situational slice of time. If the meeting goes well, your job may become less stressful, but for now, let's just focus on the meeting itself. If you could call the shots, what would you want to be the outcome of this meeting?

P: I would like to have a concrete plan for learning new tasks at work. I want a plan that my boss and I can agree on, so that I don't have to feel so nervous when I am assigned new duties.

T: That sounds like a good desired outcome – specific and attainable. Okay, so let's work the situation backward from how we usually do, since it is a prospective CSQ. Now that you have identified the desired outcome, let's identify some behaviors and thoughts that would help you to get your desired outcome. In the first step, we describe the situation.

P: My job coach, therapist, and I will be meeting to discuss a plan for ways that I can learn new tasks. I hope that we can develop a plan for ways I can learn new tasks. Right now they just show me once, and then leave me on my own.

T: Good start. Now, let's move on to the second section. In the past you said that you become frustrated and withdraw from these conversations, because people aren't meeting your expectations. What kind of thoughts are you having when you feel like that?

P: Hmmm . . . "I shouldn't even have to tell her what I need, she should just know."

T: Is that a helpful or hurtful thought, in light of your desired outcome, which is to develop a plan for learning new tasks at work?

P: Well if I am thinking that, I don't feel like talking any more. I shut down.

T: Will "shutting down" help you to develop a plan for learning new tasks at work?

P: No, I'll just withdraw and give up.

T: What would be a more helpful thought you could have?

P: "She is trying to help me."

T: Why would that thought help you to get your desired outcome?

P: It will make me feel less nervous, and like she is on my side. I can communicate better when I think someone is trying to help me. It's just hard to think clearly that when I start feeling anxious.

T: It is difficult, but now you have a plan, so you can catch your hurtful thoughts as soon you start having them. You will be looking out for them. Let's move on to step 3: the behaviors. What kind of behavior has been troubling in past conversations with her?

P: I have a hard time processing what she is saying, thinking of what I am going to say, and trying to understand and remember the conversation all at the same time. If I don't understand something, I just zone out.

T: Sounds like withdrawing hurts your chances of getting what you want. What behaviors would help to keep from getting overwhelmed?

P: It helps when I have information written down.

T: Okay, good, so I could act as secretary during the meeting, so that you can have the main points written down – that way you can focus your resources on the conversation in the moment, and not have to worry about whether you will remember it or not.

P: That would help a lot.

T: You also mentioned having difficulty understanding what she says, and kind of zoning out. One thing that you do in therapy, that I think is very useful, is ask me questions when you haven't understood what I said or if you need clarification. Do you think that might help in this situation too?

P: Yes, I could make sure I understand what she is saying, and ask her if I am not sure about something.

T: Okay, so you said that if you start getting frustrated, you will remind yourself that she is trying to help you. You also said that you would feel less overwhelmed if you knew that I was writing things down. So those things will help to decrease your anxiety, which helps you to communicate better. Is anything missing? That is, with those alone, will you get what you want?

P: Well, I really want a plan that works for me.

T: What do we need to add to the CSQ, so that you can get the plan that you want?

P: I need to express clearly what would work for me.

T: How do you express it clearly?

P: Calm and articulately. It would help me to prepare that ahead of time and write it down.

T: Great, let's add that to behaviors! So, let's recap. If you think to yourself that your vocational coach wants to help you, ask for clarification when you don't understand something, state what you want in a calm manner, and have me write down the key points of the conversation, do you think that you'll get your desired outcome – which is to have a solid plan for you to learn new tasks at work?

P: Yes, and having the meeting planned out will make me feel better.

The meeting went according to plan, and Patrick achieved his desired outcome: a written plan to help him learn new tasks at work. Therapy with Patrick also frequently involved psychoeducation about normative social interactions and relationships. For example, Patrick inquired, "When someone asks 'How are you?', how can you tell if they really want to know how you are, or if they just mean it as a greeting?" Patrick's other inquiries were about topics such as relationship boundaries, dating etiquette, and the importance of eye contact and reciprocal conversation.

Therapy also involved teaching Patrick to advocate for himself, and to ask for help in an effective manner. This was accomplished mostly in the context of CSQs. For example, some CSQs involved telling friends, family members, or co-workers about his Asperger's disorder symptoms, and how it might impact his interactions with them. In addition, Patrick's therapist assisted in generating assertive behaviors to ask for help when he needed it (e.g., asking his boss to write down work instructions, asking a friend to explain what they meant if he did not understand). The step in the CSQs involving interpretations was often used as a point of intervention for thoughts that led to him feeling overwhelmed (e.g., "I should be able to get this. I am going to have a meltdown and humiliate myself"), and changing them to more helpful thoughts (e.g., "I am starting to feel overstimulated. I'll take a five-minute break and return to this when I don't feel overstimulated"). Patrick learned to identify the onset of physical and behavioral symptoms of anxiety as times to become cognizant of his thoughts, and change hurtful thoughts to helpful thoughts.

Patrick continued to use the skills he learned from the CSQs to improve interpersonal relationships, and as a result reported feeling less lonely and depressed. For example, in an effort to broaden his social support network, he founded a support group for adults with Asperger's disorder. He reported that founding this group improved his self-esteem, and spending time with group members added enjoyment and meaning to his life.

When Patrick's symptoms had been in remission for a substantial period of time (approximately eight weeks), it was mutually decided that Patrick would take a month's hiatus from therapy to see if his gains were maintained, and that the possibility of termination would be considered. Patrick returned for the final session, and reported that he continued to improve with regard to his anxiety and depression symptoms, and also had increased functioning in occupational and social domains. Progress in therapy was consistent, and steady gains were noted during the eight months during which therapy was conducted. When asked how Patrick felt about the termination of therapy, he said, "Well, it means changing one of my routines."

CONCLUSIONS AND FUTURE DIRECTIONS

The treatment of individuals with a dual diagnosis can be very challenging for clinicians, and at times may even appear to be an impossible task. The significant developmental delays in such individuals, particularly in the areas of social skills, communication skills, and intellectual functioning present numerous challenges in the areas of assessing, diagnosing, and treatment. Research has consistently demonstrated that individuals with MR and PDDs are at greater risk for the development of psychopathology than the general population.[5-9] Also, many of these individuals may not receive a diagnosis for a variety of reasons,[15] and thus not receive the services that they need. Despite the clear need for more research in the treatment of this population, and although the field has made considerable advances in the past 20 years, there are still many questions that remain.

The purpose of this chapter was to provide information and suggestions for treating those with a dual diagnosis, as well as to review the current literature on such issues. Understanding how psychopathology is represented in individuals with MR or PDDs is the first key to treating such problems. As mentioned above, there is strong reason to believe that the current criteria in DSM-IV may need modification to be appropriate for those with MR and PDDs.[29] Unfortunately, thus far, little research has been conducted with modified diagnostic criteria for individuals with MR or PDDs. Studies have demonstrated that clients with MR and PDDs tend to display more behavioral difficulties than those without a disability, but little research exists in examining these behaviors in relation to diagnostic symptomatology of psychiatric disorders. Thus, research should focus on examining the differences in symptoms of psychopathology in individuals with MR and PDDs. Clinicians would particularly benefit from research that specifies ways to determine if an individual's behavior is "abnormal" for someone who has a developmental disability versus simply discrepant from the general population. Proper diagnosis is essential for effective treatment planning, and should therefore be made a priority in the field.

Due to the lack of such research, clinicians are often left relying on clinical intuition when determining if a comorbid diagnosis exists in individuals with PDDs. When considering the diagnosis of a comorbid psychiatric disorder, taking a developmental psychopathology approach may be very useful, such that one should consider the presence, persistence, pervasiveness, and impairment of such symptoms in the context of developmental processes. That is, the clinician should determine if the presenting behaviors and symptoms are "abnormal" in light of the individual's current developmental level rather than chronological age. Other parameters of abnormality, such as distress and impairment, are best assessed using multiple methods and informants. A multi-method multi-informant approach to assessment basically states that clinicians should use a variety of assessment methods (i.e., rating scales, interviews, functional assessments) and collect information from multiple sources close to the client. Consensus in the field is that this is not only recommended, but a necessity when assessing individuals with PDDs.

Although numerous measures have been developed to aid in the diagnosis of psychiatric disorders in populations with MR, little empirical research has been conducted on the clinical utility of such measures. Reviews of such instruments have come to the conclusion that many of these measures' psychometric properties have not been tested thoroughly and tend to have a limited range of content.[27,35] Furthermore, as with many forms of assessment, the incremental validity of such measures is largely unknown. That is, to what extent does the assessment instrument add to the treatment of individuals with PDDs? Thus, research needs to focus not on developing new instruments to measure psychopathology in this population, but rather more extensive research on the psychometric properties and clinical utility of existing instruments.

It has been suggested that functional assessment techniques and observations, including the use of behavioral descriptive instruments, are essential in the diagnosis of comorbid psychiatric disorders in clients with MR.[29,36] An interesting line of research that should be continued is the operationalizing of constructs such as happiness in terms of behaviors present in those with MR or PDDs. The work by Green and Reid,[37] as well as others, that the observation of simple behaviors, such as frequency of smiling and laughing, is a valid means of measuring happiness in individuals with PDDs, represents a significant advance in the ability to assess symptoms of psychopathology. Further advances in such areas will undoubtedly be beneficial in assessing and treating those with a dual diagnosis.

Regarding treatment, some case studies have been published in which individuals with developmental disabilities have benefited from empirically supported treatments (e.g., exposure, cognitive-behavioral therapy) that have been tested on the general population.[48,49,55] These preliminary data suggest that other empirically supported treatments might also be effective in individuals with developmental disabilities. The field of mental health would benefit greatly from large clinical trials testing out the use of empirically supported treatments with samples of individuals with developmental disabilities, since they are typically excluded from randomized trials. Rigorous scientific studies are needed in this area, so that this underserved population can receive the services they need. Obstacles involved in this type of research have been mentioned and are noteworthy, but are by no means insurmountable.

CHAPTER 8

CHAPTER 8

The Delivery of Mental Health Services for Clients of Diverse Backgrounds: Summary and Future Directions

Lora Rose Hunter, Julia D Buckner, Jill M Holm-Denoma, and Yezzennya Castro

We hope that this book will serve as a comprehensive therapeutic reference for clinicians as well as a source of future research direction for all psychologists. The authors of this book have detailed techniques therapists can use to strive for culturally competent assessment, diagnosis, and treatment of clients from diverse backgrounds. By providing a comprehensive consolidation of the existing literature, the authors have identified numerous areas in which more must be done to improve the accessibility and quality of mental health care for an increasingly diverse population.

Sue's[1] conceptualization of cultural competence has provided a simple yet effective framework for providing mental health services in a culturally sensitive and scientific way. By documenting the manner in which the clinicians at our outpatient community clinic have incorporated this framework into clinical practice, we hope to have provided the reader with clinical evidence of the importance of being knowledgeable about the common practices, experiences, and worldviews of the various cultural groups to which clients belong. This knowledge is integral as it allows the clinician to test hypotheses about the influence of cultural variables, rather than making uninformed assumptions about clients. The chapters in this book have also emphasized the importance of considering how a clinician's own culture and beliefs may affect their interpretations of clients' behavior. By making the effort to acquire culture-specific expertise, and exercising scientific mindedness and dynamic sizing, clinicians' interactions with clients will be guided by science and influenced by an appreciation for the diversity of ways in which individuals experience the world and themselves.

This final chapter will review major findings regarding assessment, diagnosis, and treatment of all clients. In addition, this chapter will discuss future directions for clinicians and researchers in critical areas relevant to individuals from all diverse backgrounds.

ASSESSMENT

As discussed throughout the book, mental health professionals should approach assessment from the stance of *scientific mindedness*.[1] With each new client, the diagnostician should develop empirically based hypotheses regarding ways in which the client's culture may or may not affect the assessment process. Furthermore, mental health professionals working within a framework of cultural competency may find it necessary to supplement their usual assessment instruments to gather additional relevant data to make informed hypotheses. To illustrate, as discussed by Brown and Van Orden in Chapter 5, the assessor may want to include a spiritual history[2,3] or spiritual assessment[4] to assess clients' levels of identification and involvement with a religious or spiritual tradition. This information can be useful in many ways, including determining whether a client's religious and/or spiritual practices are deviant (relative to others who share the same beliefs and practices) and whether religious and/or spiritual practices can be used to augment the therapeutic process (e.g., by providing social support[5]). Similarly, for some clients, it may be beneficial and necessary to assess such factors as acculturation, acculturative stress, cultural conflicts, immigration history, minority status and experiences with discrimination.[6-9] Assessment of these variables could provide valuable information regarding protective factors (e.g., family network) in addition to specific information regarding stressors that may be relevant to the etiology and/ or maintenance of psychopathology for that particular client.

Language is another important factor that should be considered by mental health professionals striving to conduct culturally competent assessments. For instance, as discussed by Jakobsons and Buckner in Chapter 2, when assessing Hispanic/Latino clients, clinicians should ascertain the language in which the client prefers the assessment be conducted. Language can affect the communication of symptomatology, leading to potentially faulty conclusions if clients are unable to clearly communicate their experiences. Thus, assessing a client's preferred language will inform which assessment measures are most appropriate for that particular client. If the client prefers the assessment be conducted in Spanish, for example, then the diagnostician must choose instruments that have demonstrated adequate psychometric properties when administered in Spanish. Additionally, if the therapist is not proficient in Spanish, they might consider using an interpreter or referring the client to a therapist who is bilingual.

Related to the issue of language, it is vital that clinicians carefully consider the phrasing of questions posed to gather assessment data. Mental health professionals need to be mindful of assumptions they may make about a particular client's cultural background and the ways in which these assumptions may be unwittingly communicated to the client. For instance, as discussed by Gordon and Castro in Chapter 4, when conducting a mental health assessment, it is recommended that the assessor does not make assumptions about the client's sexual orientation. In this example, it is recommended that the therapist ask the client whether she is currently involved in a romantic relationship rather than asking if she has a boyfriend. By striving to use neutral, unassuming language, the mental health professional can create an atmosphere in which clients do not feel they need to combat preconceived notions held by the mental health professional.

Schlauch, Gordon, and Schmidt in Chapter 7 presented some ways in which human judgment and inference is frequently flawed. As such, clinicians' judgments about clients could affect important aspects of the therapy process, including assessment. Therefore, the scientifically minded clinician will attempt to minimize the influence of human judgment on data collected during the assessment process by relying on a wide variety of symptom measures. Although the clinician will consider their and the client's interpretation of behaviors and symptoms, these interpretations should be verified using information from other sources, including perceptions of significant others, and, objective, empirically developed measures of symptomatology and behavior. This practice ensures that decisions are made based on data that converge to support a particular diagnostic impression, rather than relying solely on the clinician's judgment to make decisions about a client's behavior and symptomatology.

The delivery of culturally competent assessment procedures is not easy. In their comprehensive case example (Chapter 4), Gordon and Castro made apparent several pitfalls that can be avoided by practicing dynamic sizing. For instance, the therapist was given facts that he could have interpreted using his knowledge of stereotypes about gay men. Rather than reacting, based on these stereotypes, the therapist developed alternative hypotheses regarding the client's behavior. The therapist approached the client with these hypotheses, providing the client with the opportunity to agree or disagree with them. By avoiding assumptions and maintaining an awareness of his own beliefs and stereotypes about individuals with nonheterosexual orientations, the therapist preserved the therapeutic relationship and engaged the client in therapy instead of alienating a client who already had reservations about therapy.

DIAGNOSIS

Clinicians should also strive to apply Sue's[1] factors of cultural competence to the area of diagnosis. One way to acquire culture-specific expertise in diagnoses is to use the empirical literature to gather information about cultural differences in base rates of disorders. For instance, the results of a community-based study suggest that the prevalence of night eating syndrome (a proposed disorder that is defined by a delayed circadian shift of eating[10]) may be higher in African American women than in Caucasian women.[11] Clinicians who are culturally competent may be better able to use base rates when predicting the likelihood that clients from particular racial groups are suffering from a given disorder.

Another way clinicians can demonstrate culture-specific expertise is by becoming aware of any diagnostic features that may differ across cultures. For example, as noted in Chapter 3 by Hollar *et al.*, African American individuals who suffer from major depressive disorder (MDD) are less likely to report pessimism, self-blame, and suicidal ideation than Caucasians with the same disorder.[12] Instead, African American patients are more likely to present with complaints about other common symptoms, especially appetite changes and sleep disturbances.[12] This type of knowledge can help clinicians identify, and thus correctly treat syndromes that may present themselves slightly differently across cultural groups.

Learning about the cultural background of their clients is a fundamental way clinicians can develop culture-specific expertise. One way to accomplish this task is by encouraging clinicians to familiarize themselves with readings pertinent to the culture of interest, and to talk with other individuals from that culture to get a sense of primary values and traditions of the cultural group. In addition, clinicians should simply *ask* clients about their cultural backgrounds. Given that within-group variance is often greater than between-group variance,[13] the importance of asking one's client about their individual experience in a cultural group cannot be overstated.

As recommended by Sue,[1] clinicians should also strive to exhibit scientific mindedness when approaching the task of diagnosing a client. This can be accomplished by using scientific principles to establish a working hypothesis about their client's diagnosis, and using objective data to evaluate whether their hypothesis has been supported. For instance, as noted by Brown and Van Orden (Chapter 5), if a clinician is trying to decide whether a client meets criteria for obsessive-compulsive disorder or if the client is simply exhibiting behaviors (e.g., frequent praying) that are often experienced by individuals in the client's religious group, it is best for the clinician to apply the principles of the scientific method. Specifically, the clinician may compare the frequency and intensity of the client's behaviors with those behaviors exhibited by others with a similar religious orientation to determine whether they are abnormal by the religious group's standards. The clinician should also attempt to determine empirically whether a client's behaviors are causing him or her impairment or distress. In sum, clinicians using scientific mindedness to gather data for the purpose of diagnostic decisions will be less likely to make mistakes based on conscious or unconscious stereotypes.

In addition to cultural competence and culture-specific expertise, clinicians should engage in the practice of dynamic sizing when providing diagnostic feedback to a client. For instance, as suggested by Tannenbaum *et al.* in Chapter 6, when working with a child being cared for by an extended family (as is common in many cultural groups), the clinician may exhibit dynamic sizing by making it a priority to give diagnostic feedback to all of the child's caretakers rather than providing feedback solely to the child's parents. In addition, clinicians may present diagnostic feedback in a culturally sensitive way by considering the cultural circumstances of their clients. For example, if a clinician is seeing a client who has endorsed a homosexual preference, and the clinician believes that a diagnosis of MDD is warranted, the clinician may want to specifically tell the client that a diagnosis of MDD is unrelated to the client's sexual orientation (if this is the case with that particular client), and rather reflects a pattern of depressive symptomatology which includes sadness, anhedonia, sleep and eating dysregulation, suicidal ideation, etc. Engaging in practices such as these will likely help to build rapport between the client and therapist, and ensure that clients get proper information that is fundamental to their diagnosis and treatment.

TREATMENT

High-quality assessment and diagnosis is of the utmost importance because it informs treatment selection. Therefore, in order to determine which empirically supported treatment will be the most effective for the client's diagnosis, it is necessary to use the recommended assessment and diagnostic techniques.[14] Although it has been suggested that it may be necessary to develop particular treatments for particular groups of individuals, the extant data do not support this claim. For instance, as discussed by Jakobsons and Buckner in Chapter 2, current data do not support the superiority of treatments designed specifically for particular Hispanic/Latino populations.[15] In fact, the existing literature, albeit limited, suggests that Hispanic/Latino clients respond to traditional cognitive behavioral therapies (CBT) as well as non-Hispanic/Latino Caucasian clients for depression and anxiety.[16,17] In addition, African American clients appear to respond similarly to non-Hispanic/Latino Caucasian clients in the treatment of anxiety and depression.[18,19]

What accounts for the apparent lack of differential treatment outcomes between individuals from diverse backgrounds? As discussed in several chapters throughout this book (e.g., Chapters 2, 4), it may be that empirically supported treatments are client driven and address basic human processes which make them effective across a variety of cultural backgrounds. For instance, CBT is concerned with the identification and changing of maladaptive cognitions.[20] These goals are achieved in large part by encouraging clients to collect data to challenge cognitions within their own lives. Although individual clients may differ in the origin or content of maladaptive cognitions, the process of identifying and challenging maladaptive cognitions appears, thus far, to be universally effective. Similarly, Interpersonal Psychotherapy (IPT) and Cognitive Behavioral Analysis System of Psychotherapy (CBASP) emphasize interpersonal relationships.[21,22] In both IPT and CBASP, the client chooses interpersonal situations on which to focus. Thus, the client's values, not those of the therapist or the majority culture, dictate the direction of these treatments.

CBASP in particular is a model of treatment driven by the client's values. Specifically, the goal of CBASP is to teach the client skills to identify and obtain desired outcomes in interpersonal interactions. The desired outcome is generated by the client, and consequently is within their cultural framework. In addition, maladaptive thoughts and behaviors that thwarted the client's achievement of the desired outcome are identified by the client. Finally, these thoughts and behaviors are remediated by the client to increase the likelihood the client will obtain desired outcomes. Again, because the remediated thoughts and behaviors originate from the client, they are likely to be consistent with their cultural context.

CONCLUSIONS AND FUTURE DIRECTIONS

Because individuals from diverse populations are widely represented as clients in practices across the country, it is imperative for clinicians to be trained in culturally competent delivery of mental health services. For instance, in a survey of therapists, most report having at least one lesbian, gay, or bisexual (LGB) client.[23] Similarly, according to a national survey, at least 50% of clients believe religious/spiritual activities are beneficial to their mental heath.[24] Therapists must be familiar and comfortable with the diversity of lifestyle and thought that is present in the populations they serve. At the same time, mental health services can only help clients who are able to access high quality mental health care. Unfortunately, as mentioned in the introduction to this book, current information suggests some minority groups are much less likely to receive mental health services than majority group members, and that services they do receive are of poorer quality than those of majority group consumers.[25] This disparity is especially pronounced for the African American and Hispanic/Latino population.[26,27] By identifying reasons for underutilization of mental health services, suggestions for ways to overcome these barriers can be formulated.

The main reasons identified by earlier chapters for discrepancies in mental heath services are both economic and psychosocial. African American and Hispanic/Latino people have disproportionately low socioeconomic status (SES), which frequently includes being without health insurance. Although many places, especially university clinics, offer mental health services on a sliding cost scale or at extremely reduced rates, the community at large is not necessarily aware that affordable therapy is even an option. To reach some underserved populations, it may be necessary for mental health professionals to advertise in less traditional ways. For example, one might consider using advertisement space in smaller local publications with large minority readership rates. In addition, by allying with community centers, places of worship and charitable organizations that are well-established in poverty-stricken neighborhoods, clinicians can reach less fortunate potential consumers who might not otherwise encounter information about mental health services.

Even when people are cognizant of mental health options, cultural attitudes and beliefs about therapy may affect both their likelihood of choosing to pursue a course of psychotherapy and/or the treatment outcome. For example, in Chapter 3, Hollar *et al.* presented evidence that African American people may be hesitant to seek professional help for a variety of reasons including fears of racism, mistrust of non-African American therapists, and cultural beliefs about the appropriateness of therapy. In addition, studies indicate that individuals from underserved ethnic minority groups who seek professional help are less likely to stay in treatment and less likely to adhere to treatment requirements.[28,29] An increased presence of clinicians in ethnic minority communities could help to diminish negative attitudes towards psychotherapy. Further, by acknowledging the very real concerns of ethnic and racial minority clients, and by implementing Sue's[1] factors of culture-specific expertise (dynamic sizing, and scientific mindedness) in all areas of treatment, clinicians will likely increase the compliance and success of individuals from diverse backgrounds. Clients who experience success despite these concerns may be the primary catalyst for changing attitudes in broader community contexts.

Mental health service delivery to members of underserved and understudied cultural groups may also be improved by placing an emphasis on delivering culturally sensitive and competent services in continuing education classes. These classes would serve several functions. First, they would provide an excellent psychoeducation forum for clinicians. Second, they would help to ensure that all clients receive mental health services from professionals who have been trained in the delivery of services to diverse populations. Finally, they may help individuals in the mental health service field who possess unhelpful and/or unfair stereotypes about members from various cultural groups to overcome their biases.

The structure and content of these continuing education courses could take many forms. It may be ideal to have clinicians first presented with empirically based literature findings (much like those that are presented in this book) that inform assessment, diagnosis, and treatment. Subsequently, members from the cultural groups of interest may present personal information that will give clinicians a qualitative feeling for some of the important traditions and values of various cultures. Finally, clinicians should be taught characteristics that are relevant to the provision of mental health services with individuals from *any* cultural group, namely respect and empathy.

In addition to being respectful and empathetic of their clients, effective clinicians deliver treatments informed by empirically based literature. However, many study samples do not include significant representation of diverse populations. In the future, researchers and clinicians should make a greater effort to increase minority enrollment when standardizing assessment tools and conducting treatment efficacy studies. If cultural differences are hypothesized, the inclusion of appropriate numbers of members from diverse populations will allow for the examination of moderation and mediation effects of diversity factors.

In some cases, researchers have found that therapeutic techniques that were designed and evaluated on primarily non-Hispanic/Latino Caucasian samples are largely applicable to clients of diverse backgrounds (to illustrate, see discussion of CBT above). At the same time, some techniques are based on assumptions that limit their application. For example, as indicated in Chapter 7, the *Diagnostic and Statistical Manual of Mental Disorders*, fourth edition DSM-IV criteria for most diagnoses assume developmental normality and are not necessarily applicable to individuals with significant developmental delay. Researchers must be careful not to make assumptions about the usefulness or uselessness of assessments, diagnoses, and empirically based treatments in diverse populations. If studies include diverse samples but make erroneous assumptions, it will likely adversely affect analysis and interpretation. Similarly, studies that do not have representative samples, but use techniques that have been empirically validated in diverse groups, should be considered for broader interpretation.

The only way the field will be able to advance the delivery of mental heath services to diverse populations is by conducting investigations that include culture-specific expertise. It is clear as a result of the literature reviews in this book that there are little empirical data to this end. Two areas of particular interest for future research assessing diverse populations are differential risk and protective factors. It is known that certain factors including SES and particular life stressors contribute to a higher risk of mental illness for diverse populations, whereas other factors, such as familial organization, may protect individuals from mental illness. However, the mechanisms by which these factors result in mental illness are not well explored. Further investigation of differential risk and protective factors would allow clinicians to develop more effective prevention programs and treatments. For instance, Gordon and Castro (Chapter 4) described that LGB individuals' risk for mental illness likely results from life stressors associated with societal stigma. A better understanding of the complicated process of "coming out," as well as discrimination and prejudice, would help mental health providers tailor cognitive behavioral therapies for LGB individuals. In sum, future research is critical. We must strive to provide empirical data that will aid psychologists and clinicians in increasing access and effectiveness of treatment for the established and growing population of individuals of diverse backgrounds.

Endnotes

Notes to Chapter 1: Mental Health Services for Diverse Populations

1 Bernstein R. US Bureau of the Census. *Hispanic and Asian Americans Increasing Faster than Overall Population* [monograph on the Internet]. Washington, DC: US Bureau of the Census; 2004 [cited April 30, 2005]. Available from: www.census.gov/PressRelease/www/releases/archives/race/001839.html.

2 Projections of the resident population by age, sex, race, and Hispanic origin: 1999 to 2100 [monograph on the Internet]. Washington, DC: US Bureau of the Census; 2000 [cited April 30, 2005]. Available from: www.census.gov/population/projections/nation/detail/d2001_10.pdf.

3 State and country quick facts [homepage on the Internet]. Washington, DC: US Bureau of the Census; 2000 [last updated January 12, 2006; cited February 19, 2006]. Available from http://quickfacts.census.gov/qfd/states/00000.html.

4 American Psychological Association. Guidelines on multicultural education, training, research, practice, and organizational change for psychologists. *Am Psychol.* 2002; **58**(5): 377–402.

5 Smith DM, Gates G. *Gay and Lesbian Families in the United States* [monograph on the Internet]. Washington, DC: Urban Institute; 2001 [cited April 30, 2005]. Available from: www.urban.org/publications/1000491.html.

6 Waldrop J, Stern SM. US Disability status: 2000 [monograph on the Internet]. Washington, DC: United States Bureau of the Census; 2003 [cited April 30, 2005]. Available from: www.census.gov/prod/2003pubs/c2kbr-17.pdf.

7 Lugaila T, Overturf J. *Children and the Households They Live In* [monograph on the Internet]. Washington, DC: US Bureau of the Census; 2004 [cited 2005 April 30]. Available from: www.census.gov/prod/2004pubs/censr-14.pdf.

8 Kosmin BA, Mayer E, Keysar A. American religious identity survey [monograph on the Internet]. New York: City University of New York; 2001 [cited 2005 April 28]. Available from: www.gc.cuny.edu/faculty/research_studies/aris.pdf.

9 United States Department of Health and Human Services. *Mental Health: culture, race, and ethnicity – a supplement to mental health: a report of the surgeon general – executive summary.* Rockville, MD: US Department of Health and Human Services; 2001.

10 Robins LN, Heizer JE, Weissman MM *et al.* Lifetime prevalence of specific psychiatric disorders in three sites. *Arch Gen Psychiatry.* 1984; **41**(10): 949–58.

11 American Psychiatric Association. *Diagnostic and Statistical Manual of Mental Disorders*. 4th ed, text revision. Washington, DC: American Psychological Association; 2000.

12 DeAngelis T. New data on lesbian, gay, and bisexual mental health: new findings overturn previous beliefs. *Monitor Psychol* [serial on the Internet]. 2002 [cited April 30, 2005]; 33(2): [about 5 p.]. Available from: www.apa.org/monitor/feb02/newdata.html.

13 Roberts RE, Roberts CR, Chen YR. Ethnocultural differences in prevalence of adolescent depression. *Am J Community Psychol*. 1997; 25: 95–110.

14 Roberts RE, Sobhan M. Symptoms of depression in adolescence: a comparison of Anglo, African, and Hispanic Americans. *J Youth Adolesc*. 1992; 21: 639–51.

15 Associated Press. Single parents' kids found more prone to mental illness [newspaper on the Internet]. *Seattle Post Intelligencer*; January 24, 2003 [cited May 1, 2005]. Available from: http://seattlepi.nwsource.com/national/105581_medi24.shtml.

16 Holden B, Gitlesen JP. The association between severity of intellectual disability and psychiatric symptomatology. *J Intellect Disabil Res*. 2002; 48(6): 556–62.

17 Sue SL, Chu JY. The mental health of ethnic minority groups: challenges posed by the supplement to the surgeon general's report on mental health. *Cult Med Psychiatry*. 2003; 27(4): 447–65.

18 Williams DR, Neighbors HW, Jackson JS. Racial/ethnic discrimination and health: findings from community studies. *Am J Public Health*. 2003; 93(2): 200–8.

19 Eibner C, Sturm R, Greznez CR. Does relative deprivation predict the need for mental health services? *J Ment Health Policy Econ*. 2004; 7(4): 167–75.

20 Goodman E, Slap GB, Huang B. The public health impact of socioeconomic status on adolescent depression and obesity. *Am J Public Health*. 2003; 93(11): 1844–50.

21 Diaz RM, Ayala G, Bein E *et al*. The impact of homophobia, poverty, and racism on the mental health of gay and bisexual Latino men. *Am J Public Health*. 2001; 91(6): 927–32.

22 Emerson E. Poverty and children with intellectual disabilities in the world's richer countries. *J Intellect Dev Disabil*. 2004; 29(4): 319–38.

23 Pilkington NW, D'Augelli AR. Victimization of lesbian, gay, and bisexual youth in community settings. *J Community Psychol*. 1995; 23(1): 34–56.

24 Coll CG, Garrido M. Minorities in the United States: sociocultural context for mental health and developmental psychopathology. In: Sameroff AJ, Lewis M, Miller SM, editors. *Handbook of Developmental Psychopathology*. 2nd ed. New York: Kluwer Academic/Plenum Publishers; 2002. p. 177–95.

25 Hall GCN. Psychotherapy research with ethnic minorities: empirical, ethical, and conceptual issues. *J Consult Clin Psychol*. 2001; 69(3): 502–10.

26 Sue S. In search of cultural competence in psychotherapy and counseling. *Am Psychol*. 1998; 53(4): 440–8.

27 Sue DW, Bernier JB, Durran M *et al*. Position paper: cross-cultural counseling competencies. *Couns Psychol*. 1982; **10**: 45–52.

Notes to Chapter 2: Hispanic/Latino Clients

1 US Census Bureau. *The Hispanic Population: 2000*. Washington, DC: Government Printing Office; 2001.

2 Anthony JC, Petronix KR. Suspected risk factors for depression among adults 18–44 years old. *Epidemiology*. 1991; **2**: 123–32.

3 Kessler RC, McGonagle KA, Zhao S *et al*. Lifetime and 12-month prevalence of DSM-III-R psychiatric disorders in the United States: results from the national comorbidity study. *Arch Gen Psychiatry*. 1994; **51**: 8–19.

4 Golding JM, Karno M, Rutter CM. Symptoms of major depression among Mexican-Americans and non-Hispanic whites. *Am J Psychiatry*. 1990; **147**: 861–6.

5 US Census Bureau. *Overview of Race and Hispanic Origin: 2000*. Washington, DC: Government Printing Office; 2001.

6 Ramirez RR, de la Cruz GP. *The Hispanic Population in the United States: March 2002*. Current Population Reports. Washington, DC: Census Bureau; 2002.

7 Cuéllar I, Roberts RE. Relations of depression, acculturation and socioeconomic status in a Latino sample. *Hisp J Behav Sci*. 1997; **19**: 230–8.

8 Vega WA, Warheit G, Buhl-Auth J *et al*. The prevalence of depressive symptoms among Mexican Americans and Anglos. *Am J Epidemiol*. 1984; **120**: 592–607.

9 Hovey JD, King CA. Acculturative stress, depression, and suicidal ideation among immigrant and second-generation Latino adolescents. *J Am Acad Child Adolesc Psychiatry*. 1996; **35**: 1183–92.

10 Berry JW. Psychology of acculturation. In: Berman JJ, editor. *Cross-Cultural Perspectives*. Nebraska Symposium on Motivation; 1990 37. Lincoln, NE: University of Nebraska Press; 1990. p. 201–34.

11 Williams CL, Berry JW. Primary prevention of acculturative stress among refugees: application of psychological theory and practice. *Am Psychol*. 1991; **46**: 632–41.

12 Hovey JD. Acculturative stress, depression, and suicidal ideation in Mexican immigrants. *Cultur Divers Ethnic Minor Psychol*. 2000; **6**: 134–51.

13 Pole N, Best SR, Metzler T *et al*. Why are Hispanics at greater risk for PTSD? *Cultur Divers Ethnic Minor Psychol*. 2005; **11**: 144–61.

14 Minsky S, Vega W, Miskimen T *et al*. Diagnostic patterns in Latino, African American, and European American psychiatric patients. *Arch Gen Psychiatry*. 2003; **60**: 637–44.

15 Vega WA, Kolody B, Aguilar-Gaxiola S *et al*. Gaps in services utilization by Mexican Americans with mental health problems. *Am J Psychiatry*. 1999; **156**: 928–34.

16 Miranda J, Cooper LA. Disparities in care for depression among primary care patients. *J Gen Intern Med.* 2004; **19**: 120–6.

17 Sanchez AR, Atkinson DR. Mexican-American cultural commitment, preference for counselor ethnicity, and willingness to use counseling. *J Couns Psychol.* 1983; **30**: 215–20.

18 Brown ER, Ojeda VD, Wyn R et al. *Racial and Ethnic Disparities in Access to Health Insurance and Health Care.* Los Angeles, CA: UCLA Center for Health Policy Research and Kaiser Family Foundation; 2000.

19 Sue S. In search of cultural competence in psychotherapy and counseling. *Am Psychol.* 1998; **53**: 440–8.

20 Butcher JN, Dahlstrom WG, Graham JR et al. *Minnesota Multiphasic Personality Inventory-2 (MMPI-2): manual for administration and scoring.* Minneapolis, MN: University of Minnesota Press; 1989.

21 Hall GC, Bansal A, Lopez IR. Ethnicity and psychopathology: a meta-analytic review of 31 years of comparative MMPI/MMPI-2 Research. *Psychol Assess.* 1999; **11**: 186–97.

22 Sheldon K, Williams G, Joiner TE. Self-determination theory in the clinic. New Haven, CT: Yale University Press; 2003.

23 Butler G. Phobic disorders. In: Hawton K, Salkovskis PM, Kirk J et al., editors. *Cognitive Behavior Therapy for Psychiatric Problems: a practical guide.* New York: Oxford University Press; 1989. p. 97–128.

24 Klerman GL, Weissman MM, Rounsaville BJ et al. *Interpersonal Psychotherapy of Depression.* New York: Basic Books; 1984.

25 McCullough J. *Treatment for Chronic Depression: Cognitive Behavioral Analysis System of Psychotherapy (CBASP).* New York: Guilford Press; 2000.

26 Espinoza G, Elizondo V, Miranda J. *Hispanic Churches in American Public Life: summary of findings.* (Interim Rep. No. 2). Notre Dame, IN: University of Notre Dame, Institute for Latino Studies; 2003.

27 American Psychological Association. Guidelines for providers of psychological services to ethnic, linguistic, and culturally diverse populations. *Am Psychol.* 1993; **48**: 45–8.

28 Alvidrez J, Azocar F, Miranda J. Demystifying the concept of ethnicity for psychotherapy researchers. *J Consult Clin Psychol.* 1996; **64**: 903–8.

29 Altarriba J, Santiago-Rivera AL. Current perspectives on using linguistic and cultural factors in counseling the Hispanic client. *Prof Psychol Res Pr.* 1994; **25**: 388–97.

30 Hall GC. Psychotherapy research with ethnic minorities: empirical, ethical, and conceptual issues. *J Consult Clin Psychol.* 2001; **69**: 502–10.

31 Rogler LH, Cortes DE, Malgady RG. Acculturation and mental health status among Hispanics. *Am Psychol.* 1991; **46**: 585–97.

32 Escobar JI, Nervi CH, Gara MA. Immigration and mental health: Mexican Americans in the United States. *Harv Rev Psychiatry.* 2000; **8**: 64–72.

33 Rodriguez N, Myers HF, Mira CB *et al*. Development of the multidimensional acculturative stress inventory for adults of Mexican origin. *Psychol Assess*. 2002; **14**: 451–61.

34 Cervantes RC, Padilla AM, de Snyder NS. The Hispanic stress inventory: a culturally relevant approach to psychosocial assessment. *J Consult Clin Psychol*. 1991; **3**: 438–47.

35 Rodriguez-Gomez JR, Caban M. The problem of bilingualism in psychiatric diagnoses of Hispanic clients. *Cross-Cult Psychol Bull*. 1992; **26**: 2–5.

36 Marcos LR, Alpert M, Urcuyo L *et al*. The effect of interview language on the evaluation of psychopathology in Spanish-American schizophrenic patients. *Am J Psychiatry*. 1973; **130**: 549–53.

37 Guttfreund DG. Effects of language usage on emotional experience of Spanish-English and English-Spanish bilinguals. *J Consult Clin Psychol*. 1990; **58**: 604–7.

38 Marcos LR. Bilinguals in psychotherapy: language as an emotional barrier. *Am J Psychother*. 1976; **30**: 552–60.

39 Vasquez JN, Javier RA. The problem with interpreters: communicating with Spanish-speaking patients. *Hosp Community Psychiatry*. 1991; **42**: 163–5.

40 Brislin RW. *Understanding Culture's Influence on Behavior*. New York: Harcourt Brace Jovanisch; 1993.

41 First MB, Spitzer RL, Gibbon M *et al*. *Entrevista Clínica Estructurada Para los Trastornos del eje I del DSM-IV, Versión Clónica*. Barcelona, Spain: Masson; 1999.

42 First MB, Gibbon M, Spitzer RL *et al*. *Entrevista clónica Estructurada Para los Trastornos de Personalidad del eje II del DSM-IV*. Barcelona, Spain: Masson; 1999.

43 Karno M, Burnam A, Escobar JL *et al*. Development of the national institute of mental health diagnostic interview schedule. *Arch Gen Psychiatry*. 1983; **40**: 1183–8.

44 Haslin D, Trautman K, Miele G *et al*. *Psychiatric Research Interview for Substance and Mental Disorders (PRISM)*. New York: New York State Psychiatric Institute/ Columbia University; 1995.

45 Beck A, Steer RA. *Beck Anxiety Inventory Manual*. San Antonio, TX: Psychological Corporation; 1990.

46 Beck A, Steer R, Brown G. *Beck Depression Inventory, Second Edition Manual*. San Antonio, TX: Psychological Corporation; 1996.

47 Beck A. *Beck Depression Inventory: Spanish translation*. San Antonio, TX: Psychological Corporation; 1993.

48 Beck A, Epstein N, Brown G *et al*. An inventory for measuring clinical anxiety properties. *J Consult Clin Psychol*. 1998; **56**: 893–7.

49 Garner DM, Olmstead MP, Polivy J. Development and validation of a multidimensional eating disorder inventory for anorexia nervosa and bulimia. *Int J Eat Disord*. 1983; **2**: 15–34.

50 Machado PPP, Goncalves S, Martins C *et al*. The Portuguese version of the eating disorders inventory: evaluation of its psychometric properties. *Eur Eat Disord Rev*. 2001; **9**: 43–52.

51 Azocar F, Areán P, Miranda J et al. Differential item functioning in a Spanish translation of the Beck depression inventory. J Clin Psychol. 2001; 57: 355–65.

52 Padilla ER, Olmedo EL, Loya F. Acculturation and the MMPI performance of Chicano and Anglo college students. Hisp J Behav Sci. 1982; 4: 451–66.

53 Whitworth R. Anglo- and Mexican-American performance on the MMPI administered in Spanish or English. J Clin Psychol. 1988; 44: 891–7.

54 Montgomery GT, Orozco S. Mexican-Americans' performance on the MMPI as a function of level of acculturation. J Clin Psychol. 1983; 41: 208–12.

55 Contreras S, Fernandez S, Malcarne VL et al. Reliability and validity of the Beck depression and anxiety inventories in Caucasian Americans and Latinos. Hisp J Behav Sci. 2004; 26: 446–62.

56 Gray-Little B. The assessment of psychopathology in racial and ethnic minorities. In: Butcher J, editor. Clinical Personality Assessment: practical approaches. 2nd edition. New York: Oxford University Press; 2002. p. 171–89.

57 Roberts E, Chen Y. Depressive symptoms and suicidal ideation among Mexican-origin and Anglo adolescents. J Am Acad Child Adolesc Psychiatry. 1995; 34: 81–90.

58 Escobar JI. Transcultural aspects of dissociative and somatoform disorders. Psychiatr Clin North Am. 1995; 18: 555–69.

59 Maercker A, Herrle J. Long-term effects of the Dresden bombing: relationships to control beliefs, religious belief, and personal growth. J Trauma Stress. 2003; 16: 579–87.

60 Potter LB, Rogler LH, Moscicki EK. Depression among Puerto Ricans in New York City: the Hispanic health and nutrition examination survey. Soc Psychiatry Psychiatr Epidemiol. 1995; 30: 185–93.

61 Narrow WE, Rae DS, Moscicki EK et al. Depression among Cuban Americans: the Hispanic health and nutrition survey. Soc Psychiatry Psychiatr Epidemiol. 1990; 25: 260–8.

62 Burnam MR, Hough J, Escobar M et al. Six-month prevalence of specific psychiatric disorders among Mexican American and non-Hispanic whites in Los Angeles. Arch Gen Psychiatry. 1987; 44: 687–94.

63 Karno M, Hough RL, Burnam MA et al. Lifetime prevalence of specific psychiatric disorders among Mexican Americans and non-Hispanic whites in Los Angeles. Arch Gen Psychiatry. 1987; 44: 695–701.

64 Vega WA, Kolody B, Aguilar-Goxiola S et al. Lifetime prevalence of DSM-III-R psychiatric disorders among urban and rural Mexican Americans in California. Arch Gen Psychiatry. 1998; 55: 771–8.

65 Joiner TJ, Perez M, Wagner K.D. et al. On fatalism, pessimism, and depressive symptoms among Mexican-American and other adolescents attending an obstetrics-gynecology clinic. Behav Res Ther. 2001; 39: 887–96.

66 American Psychiatric Association. Diagnostic and Statistical Manual of Mental Disorders. 4th ed. Washington, DC: American Psychiatric Association; 1994.

67 Comas-Diaz L. Effects of cognitive and behavioral group treatment on the depressive symptomatology of Puerto Rican women. *J Consult Clin Psychol.* 1981; **49**: 627–32.

68 Miranda J, Chung JY, Green BL *et al.* Treating depression in predominantly low-income young minority women: a randomized controlled trial. JAMA 2003; **290**: 57–65.

69 Miranda J, Schoenbaum M, Sherbourne C *et al.* Effects of primary care depression treatment on minority patients' clinical status and employment. *Arch Gen Psychiatry.* 2004; **61**: 827–34.

70 Wells K, Sherbourne C, Schoenbaum M *et al.* Five-year impact of quality improvement for depression: results of a group-level randomized controlled trial. *Arch Gen Psychiatry.* 2004; **61**: 378–86.

71 Mufson L, Dorta KP, Wickramaratne P *et al.* A randomized effectiveness trial of interpersonal psychotherapy for depressed adolescents. *Arch Gen Psychiatry.* 2004; **61**: 577–84.

72 Muñoz RF, Ying YW, Pérez-Stable EJ *et al.* *The Prevention of Depression: research and practice.* Baltimore, MD: Johns Hopkins University Press; 1993.

73 Pina AA, Silverman WK, Fuentes RM *et al.* Exposure-based cognitive-behavioral treatment for phobic and anxiety disorders: treatment effects and maintenance for Hispanic/Latino relative to European-American youths. *J Am Acad Child Adolesc Psychiatry.* 2003; **42**: 1179–87.

74 Silverman WK, Kurtines WM, Ginsburg GS *et al.* Treating anxiety disorders in children with group cognitive-behavioral therapy: a randomized clinical trial. *J Consult Clin Psychol.* 1999; **67**: 995–1003.

75 Malgady RG, Rogler LH, Costantino G. Hero/heroine modeling for Puerto Rican adolescents: a preventive mental health intervention. *J Consult Clin Psychol.* 1990; **58**: 469–74.

76 Malgady RG, Rogler LH, Costantino G. Culturally sensitive psychotherapy for Puerto Rican children and adolescents: a program of treatment outcome research. *J Consult Clin Psychol.* 1990; **58**: 704–12.

77 Maramba GG, Hall GCN. Meta-analyses of ethnic match as a predictor of dropout, utilization, and level of functioning. *Cultur Divers Ethnic Minor Psychol.* 2002; **8**: 290–7.

78 Atkinson DR, Casas A, Abreu J. Mexican-American acculturation, counselor ethnicity and cultural sensitivity, and perceived counselor competence. *J Couns Psychol.* 1992; **39**: 515–20.

79 Joiner TE, Walker RL, Rudd MD *et al.* Scientizing and routinizing the assessment of suicidality in outpatient practice. *Prof Psychol Res Pr.* 1999; **30**: 1–7.

80 Beck AT, Steer RA. *Beck Scale for Suicide Ideation.* San Antonio, TX: The Psychological Corporation; 1993.

81 Sheehan DV, Lecrubier Y, Harnett-Sheehan K *et al.* Reliability and validity of the MINI international neuropsychiatric interview (MINI): according to the SCID-P. *Eur Psychiatry.* 1997; **12**: 232–41.

82 Bernal G, Bonillo J, Bellido C. Ecological validity and cultural sensitivity for outcome research for the cultural adaptation and development of psychosocial treatments with Hispanics. *J Abnorm Child Psychol*. 1995; **23**: 67–82.
83 Zuniga MA. Using metaphors in therapy: dichos and Latino clients. *Soc Work*. 1992; **37**: 55–60.
84 Galvan R, Teschner R. *El Diccionario del Español Chicano: the dictionary of Chicano Spanish*. Lincolnwood, IL: National Textbook Co; 1989.
85 Kazdin AE. Current (lack of) status of theory in child and adolescent psychotherapy research. *J Clin Child Psychol*. 1999; **28**: 533–43.

Notes to Chapter 3: African American Clients

1 Goldman HH, Rye P, Sirovatka P. *Mental Health: a report of the surgeon general*. Rockville, MD: US Department of Health and Human Services; 1999. Available from: www.surgeongeneral.gov/library/mentalhealth/home.html.
2 US Center for Mental Health Services. Cultural competence standards in managed care mental health services: Four underserved/underrepresented racial/ethnic groups. Rockville, MD: US Center for Mental Health Services; 2000.
3 Freimuth VS, Quinn SC, Thomas SB *et al*. African American individuals' views on research and the Tuskegee Syphilis Study. *Soc Sci Med*. 2001; **52**: 797–808.
4 Havassy BE, Hopkin JT. Factors predicting utilization of acute psychiatric inpatient services by frequently hospitalized patients. *Hosp Community Psychiatry*. 1989; **40**(8): 820–3.
5 Lindsey KP, Paul GL. Involuntary commitments to public mental institutions: issues involving the overrepresentation of blacks and assessment of relevant functioning. *Psychol Bull*. 1989; **106**(2): 171–83.
6 Snowden LR, Cheung FK. Use of inpatient mental health services by members of ethnic minority groups. *Am Psychol*. 1990; **45**(3): 347–55.
7 Sanchez-Hucles J. *The First Session with African-Americans: a step-by-step guide (first session)*. San Francisco, CA: Jossey-Bass; 2000.
8 Heller, J. Syphilis victims in the US study went untreated for 40 years. *The New York Times*; July 26, 1972 [cited July 20, 2005]. Available from: http://pqasb. pqarchiver.com/nytimes/80798097.html?did=80798097&FMT=ABS&FMTS=AI&date=Jul+26%2C+1972&author=By+JEAN+HELLERThe+Associated+Press&pub=New+York+Times++(1857Current+file)&desc=Syphilis+Victims+in+U.S.+Study+Went+Untreated+for+40+Years.
9 US Advisory Committee on Human Radiation Experiments, Final Report. Washington, DC: Government Printing Office; 1995.
10 Sue S, Zane N. The role of culture and cultural techniques in psychotherapy: a critique and reformulation. *Am Psychol*. 1987; **42**(1): 37–45.
11 Shavers-Hornaday V, Lynch C, Burmeister L *et al*. Why are African American individuals under-represented in medical research studies? Impediments to participation. *Ethn Health*. 1997; **2**: 31–45.

12 Ryan, RM, Deci EL. Intrinsic and extrinsic motivations: classic definitions and new directions. *Contemp Educ Psychol*. 2000; **25**: 54–67.

13 Ibrahim F, Kahn H. Assessment of worldviews. *Psychol Rep*. 1987; **60**: 163–76.

14 Morris EF. Clinical practices with African American individuals: juxtaposition of standard clinical practices and Africentricism. *Prof Psychol Res Pr*. 2001; **32**(6): 563–72.

15 Gutierrez PM, Osman A, Kopper BA *et al*. The comparative frequency of depression in various age groups. *J Gerontol*. 1976; **31**: 282–92.

16 Mezzich JE, Kleinman A, Fabrcgatt GB *et al*. Cultural proposals for DSM-IV. Pittsburgh, PA: NIMH Culture and Diagnosis Group; 1992.

17 Smith-Ruiz D. Relationship between depression, social support, and physical illness among elderly blacks: research notes. *J Natl Med Assoc*. 1985; **77**: 1017–19.

18 Butcher JN, Dahlstrom WG, Graham JR *et al*. Minnesota multiphasic personality inventory – 2 (MMPI-2): manual for administration and scoring. Minneapolis, MN: University of Minnesota Press; 1989.

19 Graham JR. *MMPI-2: Assessing Personality and Psychopathology*. 3rd ed. New York: Oxford University Press; 1999.

20 El-Sadr W, Capps L. The challenge of minority recruitment in clinical trials for AIDS. *JAMA* 1992; **267**: 954–7.

21 Freedman T. "Why don't they come to Pike street and ask us?": Black American women's health concerns. *Soc Sci Med*. 1998; **47**: 941–7.

22 Harris Y, Gorelick PH, Samuels P *et al*. Why African American individuals may not be participating in clinical trials. *J Natl Med Assoc*. 1996; **88**: 630–4.

23 Swanson G, Ward A. Recruiting minorities into clinical trials: toward a participant-friendly system. *J Natl Cancer Inst*. 1995; **87**: 1747–59.

24 Unger R, Crawford M. *Women and Gender: a feminist psychology*. 2nd ed. New York: McGraw-Hill; 1996.

25 American Psychiatric Association. *Diagnostic and Statistical Manual of Mental Disorders*. 4th ed. Washington, DC: American Psychiatric Association; 1994.

26 Devine PG, Plant EA, Buswell BN. Breaking the prejudice habit: progress and obstacles. In: Oskamp S, editor. *Reducing Prejudice and Discrimination*. Mahwah, NJ: Erlbaum; 2000. p. 185–208.

27 Kawakami K, Dovidio JF, Moll J *et al*. Just say no (to stereotyping): effects of training on the negation of stereotypic associations on stereotype activation. *J Pers Soc Psychol*. 2000; **78**: 871–88.

28 Plant EA, Devine PG. Internal and external motivation to respond without prejudice. *J Pers Soc Psychol*. 1998; **75**(3): 811–32.

29 Ashby FG, Waldron EM, Lee WW *et al*. Suboptimality in human categorization and identification. *J Exp Psychol Gen*. 2001; **130**(1): 77–96.

30 American Psychological Association. Guidelines on multicultural education, training, research, practice, and organizational change for psychologists. Washington, DC; 2002 [cited June 10, 2005]. Available from: www.apa.org/pi/multiculturalguidelines.pdf.

31 Neighbors HW, Jackson JS, Campbell L et al. The influence of racial factors on psychiatric diagnosis: a review and suggestions for research. *Community Ment Health J*. 1989; **24**: 301–11.

32 Chambless DL, Baker MJ, Baucom DH et al. Update on empirically validated therapies II. *Clin Psychol*. 1998; **51**: 3–14.

33 Lacy C, Armstrong LL, Goldman MP et al., editors. *Drug Information Handbook*, 11th ed. Hudson, OH: Lexi-Comp; 2003.

34 Svensson CK. Representation of American blacks in clinical trials of new drugs. *JAMA* 1989; **261**: 263–5.

35 Beck AT, Rush AJ, Shaw BF et al. *Cognitive Therapy of Depression*. New York: Guilford Press; 1979.

36 Dana RH. *Understanding Cultural Identity in Intervention and Assessment*. Thousand Oaks, CA: Sage; 1998.

37 McLoyd VC. Socioeconomic disadvantage and child development. *Am Psychol*. 1998; **53**: 185–204.

38 Miller WR, Rollnick S. *Motivational Interviewing: preparing people for change*. 2nd ed. New York: Guilford Press; 2002.

39 Arbisi PA, Ben-Porath YS, McNulty JL. A comparison of MMPI-2 validity in African American and Caucasian psychiatric inpatients. *Psychol Assess*. 2002; **14**: 3–15.

40 Dahlstrom WG, Lachar D, Dahlstrom LE. MMPI patterns of American minorities. Minneapolis, MN: University of Minnesota Press; 1986.

41 Hall GCN, Bansal A, Lopez IR. Ethnicity and psychopathology: a meta-analytic review of 31 years of comparative MMPI/MMPI-2 research. *Psychol Assess*. 1999; **11**(2): 186–97.

42 Timbrook RE, Graham JR. Ethnic differences on the MMPI-2? *Psychol Assess*. 1994; **6**(3): 212–17.

43 Eisen S, Dill DL, Grob MC. Reliability and validity of a brief patient report instrument for psychiatric outcome evaluation. *Hosp Community Psychiatry*. 1994; **45**: 242–7.

44 Eysenck HJ. *The Intelligence Controversy*. New York: Wiley, 1981.

45 Powers KM, Hagans-Murillo KS, Restori AF. Twenty-five years after Larry P: the California response to overrepresentation of African American individuals in special education. *Calif Sch Psychol*. 2004; **9**: 145–58.

46 Suzuki LA, Valencia RR. Race-ethnicity and measured intelligence: educational implications. *Am Psychol*. 1997; **52**(10): 1103–14.

47 Bridge GR. *The Determinants of Educational Outcomes: the impact of families, peers, teachers, and schools*. Cambridge, MA: Ballinger Publishing Co; 1979.

48 Clark R, Anderson NB, Clark VR et al. Racism as a stressor for African American individuals: a biopsychosocial model. *Am Psychol*. 1999; **54**: 805–16.

49 Borowsky SJ, Rubenstein LV, Meredith LS et al. Who is at risk of nondetection of mental health problems in primary care? *J Gen Intern Med*. 2000; **15**: 381–8.

50 Dunn LM. Special education for the mildly retarded: is much of it justifiable? *Except Child*. 1968; **23**: 5–21.

51 Finn JD. Patterns in special education placement as revealed by the OCR survey. In: Heller KA, Holtzman W, Messick S, editors. Placing children in special education: a strategy for equity. Washington, DC: National Academy Press; 1982. p. 322–81.

52 Mercer J. The pluralistic assessment project: sociocultural effects in clinical assessment. *Sch Psychol Dig.* 1973; **2**(4): 10–18.

53 Patton JM. The disproportionate representation of African American individuals in special education: looking behind the curtain for understanding and solutions. *J Spec Educ.* 1998; **32**(1): 25–31.

54 Strakowski SM, Hawkins JM, Keck PE *et al.* The effects of race and information variance on disagreement between psychiatric emergency service and research diagnoses in first-episode psychosis. *J Clin Psychiatry.* 1997; **58**: 457–63.

55 DelBello MP, Lopez-Larson MP, Soutullo CA *et al.* Effects of race on psychiatric diagnosis of hospitalized adolescents: a retrospective chart review. *J Child Adolesc Psychopharmacol.* 2001; **11**(1): 95–103.

56 Strakowski SM, Flaum M, Amador X *et al.* Racial differences in the diagnosis of psychosis. *Schizophr Res.* 1996; **21**(2): 117–24.

57 Strakowski SM, Lonczak HS, Sax KW *et al.* The effects of race on diagnosis and disposition from a psychiatric emergency service. *J Clin Psychiatry.* 1995; **56**(3): 101–7.

58 Iwamasa GY, Larrabee AL, Merritt RD. Are personality disorder criteria ethnically biased? A card-sort analysis. *Cultur Divers Ethnic Minor Psychol.* 2000; **6**(3): 284–97.

59 Gordon KH, Perez M, Joiner TE. The impact of racial stereotypes on eating disorder recognition. *Int J Eat Disord.* 2002; **32**(2): 219–24.

60 Garlow SJ, Purselle D, Heninger M. Ethnic differences in patterns of suicide across the life cycle. *Am J Psychiatry.* 2005; **162**(2): 319–23.

61 Willis LA, Coombs DW, Drentea P *et al.* Uncovering the mystery: factors of African American suicide. *Suicide Life Threat Behav.* 2003; **33**(4): 412–29.

62 Ayalon L, Young MA. A comparison of depressive symptoms in African Americans and Caucasian Americans. *J Cross Cult Psychol.* 2003; **34**(1): 111–24.

63 Jones EE. Effects of race on psychotherapy process and outcome: an exploratory investigation. *Psychother Theory Res Prac.* 1978; **15**: 226–36.

64 Matthews AK, Peterman AH. Improving provision of effective treatment for racial and cultural minorities. *Psychotherapy.* 1998; **35**: 291–305.

65 Sattler JM. The effects of therapist-client racial similarity. In: Gurman AS, Razin AM, editors. *Effective Psychotherapy: a handbook of research.* Elmsford, NY: Pergamon; 1977. p. 252–90.

66 Atkinson DR. Similarity in counseling. *Couns Psychol.* 1986; **14**: 319–54.

67 Coleman HLK, Wampold BE, Casali SL. Ethnic minorities' ratings of ethnically similar and European American counselors: a meta-analysis. *J Couns Psychol.* 1995; **42**: 55–64.

68 Erdur O, Rude SS, Baron A. Symptom improvement and length of treatment in ethnically similar and dissimilar client-therapist pairings. *J Couns Psychol*. 2003; **50**: 52–8.

69 Sue S, Fujino DC, Hu L *et al*. Community mental health services for ethnic minority groups: a test of the cultural responsiveness hypothesis. *J Consult Clin Psychol*. 1991; **59**: 533–40.

70 Miranda J, Munoz R. Intervention for minor depression in primary care patients. *Psychosom Med*. 1994; **56**: 136–41.

71 Weissman MM, Markowitz JC, Klerman GL. *Comprehensive Guide to Interpersonal Psychotherapy*. New York: Basic Books; 2000.

72 Brown C, Schulberg HC, Sacco D *et al*. Effectiveness of treatments for major depression in primary medical care practice: a post hoc analysis of outcomes for African American and white patients. *J Affect Disord*. 1999; **53**: 185–92.

73 Williams KE, Chambless DL, Steketee G. Behavioral treatment of obsessive-compulsive disorder in African-Americans: clinical issues. *J Behav Ther Exp Psychiatry*. 1998; **29**: 163–70.

74 Baker FM, Stokes-Thompson J, Davis OA *et al*. Two-year outcomes of psychosocial rehabilitation of black patients with chronic mental illness. *Psychiatr Serv*. 1999; **50**: 535–9.

75 Beck AT, Steer RA. *Beck Scale for Suicidal Ideation*. San Antonio, TX: Psychological Corporation; 1993.

76 Beck AT, Epstein N, Brown G *et al*. An inventory for measuring clinical anxiety: psychometric properties. *J Consult Clin Psychol*. 1988; **56**: 893–7.

77 Beck AT, Steer RA. *Beck Depression Inventory – Manual*. San Antonio, TX: Psychological Corporation; 1993.

78 McCullough JP. *Treatment for Chronic Depression: cognitive-behavioral analysis system of psychotherapy*. New York: Guilford Press; 2000.

Notes to Chapter 4: LGB Clients

1 Laumann EO, Gagnon JH, Michael RT *et al*. *The Social Organization of Sexuality: sexual practices in the United States*. Chicago: University of Chicago Press; 1994.

2 Kinsey AC, Pomeroy WB, Martin CE. *Sexual Behavior in the Human Male*. Oxford: Saunders; 1948.

3 Kinsey AC, Pomeroy WB, Martin CE *et al*. *Sexual Behavior in the Human Female*. Oxford: Saunders; 1953.

4 Cochran SD, Sullivan JG, Mays VM. Prevalence of mental disorders, psychological distress, and mental health services use among lesbian, gay, and bisexual adults in the United States. *J Consult Clin Psychol*. 2003; **71**: 53–61.

5 Pachankis JE, Goldfried MR. Clinical issues in working with lesbian, gay, and bisexual clients. *Psychother Theory Res Prac Train*. 2004; **41**: 227–46.

6 Garnets L, Hancock KA, Cochran SD *et al*. Issues in psychotherapy with lesbians and gay men: a survey of psychologists. *Am Psychol*. 1991; **46**: 964–72.

7   American Psychiatric Association. *Diagnostic and Statistical Manual of Mental Disorders*. 1st ed. Washington, DC: Mental Hospitals Service; 1952.

8   Association Psychiatric Association. *Diagnostic and Statistical Manual of Mental Disorders*. 2nd ed. Washington, DC: Mental Hospitals Service; 1968.

9   Hooker E. The adjustment of the male overt homosexual. *J Proj Tech*. 1957; **21**: 18–31.

10 Spitzer RL. Can some gay men and lesbians change their sexual orientation? 200 participants reporting a change from homosexual to heterosexual orientation. *Arch Sex Behav*. 2003; **32**: 403–17.

11 Bright C. Deconstructing reparative therapy: an examination of the processes involved when attempting to change sexual orientation. *Clin Soc Work J*. 2004; **32**: 471–80.

12 Haldeman DC. The practice and ethics of sexual orientation conversion therapy. *J Consult Clin Psychol*. 1994; **62**: 221–7.

13 Shidlo A, Schroeder M. Changing sexual orientation: a consumer's report. *Prof Psychol Res Prac*. 2002; **33**: 249–59.

14 Coyle A. A study of psychological well-being among gay men using the GHQ-30. *Br J Clin Psychol*. 1993; **32**(Pt 2): 218–20.

15 Herek GM. Gay people and government security clearances: a social science perspective. *Am Psychol*. 1990; **45**: 1035–42.

16 Meyer I. Prejudice, social stress, and mental health in lesbian, gay, and bisexual populations: conceptual issues and research evidence. *Psychol Bull*. 2003; **129**: 674–97.

17 Mays VM, Cochran SD. Mental health correlates of perceived discrimination among lesbian, gay, and bisexual adults in the united states. *Am J Public Health*. 2001; **91**: 1869–76.

18 Association Psychiatric Association. Guidelines for psychotherapy with lesbian, gay, and bisexual clients. *Am Psychol*. 2000; **55**: 1440–51.

19 Sue S. In search of cultural competence in psychotherapy and counseling. *Am Psychol*. 1998; **53**: 440–8.

20 Williams T, Connolly J, Pepler D *et al*. Questioning and sexual minority adolescents: high school experiences of bullying, sexual harassment and physical abuse. *Can J Community Ment Health*. 2003; **22**: 47–58.

21 Schneider MS, Brown LS, Glassgold JM. Implementing the resolution on appropriate therapeutic responses to sexual orientation: a guide for the perplexed. *Prof Psychol Res Prac*. 2002; **33**: 265–76.

22 Jones MA, Gabriel MA. Utilization of psychotherapy by lesbians, gay men, and bisexuals: findings from a nationwide survey. *Am J Orthopsychiatry*. 1999; **69**: 209–19.

23 Frank E. *Treating Bipolar Disorder: a clinician's guide to interpersonal and social rhythm therapy*. New York: Guilford Press; 2005.

24 The Kinsey Institute [homepage on the Internet]. Bloomington: The Kinsey Institute; c1996–2006 [cited 7 May, 2006]. The Kinsey Institute Library and Special Collections; [1 screen]. Available from: www.indiana.edu/~kinsey/library/.

25 Beck AT, Rush A, Shaw B. *Cognitive Therapy of Depression*. New York: Guilford Press; 1979.

26 Lewinsohn PM, Munoz RF, Youngren MA *et al*. *Control Your Depression*. Revised. New York: Simon & Schuster; 1992.

27 Barlow D. *Anxiety and Its Disorders: the nature and treatment of anxiety and panic*. New York: Guilford Press; 2002.

28 Burns DD. *Feeling Good: the new mood therapy*. New York: Harper Collins Publishers; 1998.

29 Miller WR, Rollnick S. *Motivational Interviewing: preparing people for change*. 2nd ed. New York: Guilford Press; 2002.

30 Weismann MM, Markowitz JC. *Comprehensive Guide to Interpersonal Psychotherapy*. New York: Basic Books; 2000.

31 McCullough JJ. *Treatment for Chronic Depression: cognitive behavioral analysis system of psychotherapy*. New York: Guilford Press; 2000.

32 Liszcz A, Yarhouse M. Same-sex attraction: a survey regarding client-directed treatment goals. *Psychother Theory Res Prac Train*. 2005; **42**: 111–15.

33 Lewis RJ, Derlega VJ, Clarke EG *et al*. An expressive writing intervention to cope with lesbian-related stress: the moderating effects of openness about sexual orientation. *Psychol Women Quart*. 2005; **29**: 149–57.

34 Pennebaker JW. *Writing to Heal: a guided journal for recovering from trauma and emotional upheaval*. Oakland, CA: New Harbinger Publications; 2004.

35 Kamphuis JH, Finn SE. Incorporating base rate information in daily clinical decision making. In: Butcher J, editor. *Clinical Personality Assessment: practical approaches*. 2nd ed. London: Oxford University Press; 2002. p. 256–68.

36 Carlat DJ, Camargo CA Jr, Herzog DB. Eating disorders in males: a report on 135 patients. *Am J Psychiatry*. 1997; **154**: 1127–32.

37 Kaminski PL, Chapman BP, Haynes SD *et al*. Body image, eating behaviors, and attitudes toward exercise among gay and straight men. *Eat Behav*. 2005; **6**: 179–87.

38 Russell CJ, Keel PK. Homosexuality as a specific risk factor for eating disorders in men. *Int J Eat Disord*. 2002; **31**: 300–6.

39 Austin SB, Ziyadeh N, Kahn JA *et al*. Sexual orientation, weight concerns, and eating-disordered behaviors in adolescent girls and boys. *J Am Acad Child Adolesc Psychiatry*. 2004; **43**: 1115–23.

40 Moore F, Keel P. Influence of sexual orientation and age on disordered eating attitudes and behaviors in women. *Int J Eat Disord*. 2003; **34**: 370–4.

41 Heffernan K. Eating disorders and weight concern among lesbians. *Int J Eat Disord*. 1996; **19**: 127–38.

42 van Heeringen C, Vincke J. Suicidal acts and ideation in homosexual and bisexual young people: a study of prevalence and risk factors. *Soc Psychiatry Psychiatr Epidemiol*. 2000; **35**: 494–9.

43 Wichstrom L, Hegna K. Sexual orientation and suicide attempt: a longitudinal study of the Norwegian adolescent population. *J Abnorm Psychol*. 2003; **112**: 144–51.

44 Joiner TE, Walker R, Rudd M. Scientizing and routinizing the assessment of suicidality in outpatient practice. *Prof Psychol Res Prac*. 1999; **30**: 447–53.

45 Liddle B. Therapist sexual orientation, gender, and counseling practices as they related to ratings of helpfulness by gay and lesbian clients. *J Couns Psychol*. 1996; **43**: 394–401.

46 Brooks V. Sex and sexual orientation as variables in therapists' biases and therapy outcomes. *Clin Soc Work J*. 1981; **9**: 198–210.

47 Herek G, Glunt E. Interpersonal contact and heterosexuals' attitudes toward gay men: results from a national survey. *J Sex Res*. 1993; **30**: 239–44.

48 Butcher J, Dahlstrom W, Graham J. *MMPI-2: manual for administration and scoring*. Minneapolis, MN: University of Minnesota Press; 1998.

49 Beck A, Clark D. Anxiety and depression: an information processing perspective. *Anxiety Res*. 1998; **1**: 23–6.

50 Beck A, Steer R, Brown G. *Manual for the Beck Depression Inventory-II*. San Antonio, TX: Psychological Corporation; 1996.

51 Selzer M, Vinokur A, van Rooijen L. A self-administered Short Michigan Alcoholism Screening Test (SMAST). *J Stud Alcohol*. 1975; **36**: 117–26.

52 Safren S. Affirmative, evidence-based, and ethically sound psychotherapy with lesbian, gay, and bisexual clients. *Clin Psychol Sci Prac*. 2005; **12**: 29–32.

53 Sherry A, Whilde M, Patton J. Gay, lesbian, and bisexual training competencies in American Psychological Association accredited graduate programs. *Psychother Theory Res Prac Train*. 2005; **42**: 116–20.

Notes to Chapter 5: Religiously Diverse Clients

1 Emmons RA, Paloutzian RF. The psychology of religion. *Annu Rev Psychol*. 2003; **54**: 377–402.

2 Hill PC, Pargament KI, Hood RW Jr *et al*. Conceptualizing religion and spirituality: points of commonality, points of departure. *J Theory Soc Behav*. 2000; **30**(1): 51–77.

3 Anandarajah G, Hight E. Spirituality and medical practice: using HOPE questions as a practical tool for spiritual assessment. *Am Fam Physician*. 2001; **63**(1): 81–9.

4 Richards PS, Bergin AE. Toward religious and spiritual competency for mental health professionals. In: Richards PS, Bergin AE, editors. *Handbook of Psychotherapy and Religious Diversity*. Washington, DC: American Psychological Association; 2000. p. 3–26.

5 Aponte HJ. Spirituality: the heart of therapy. *J Fam Psychother*. 2002; **13**(1): 13–27.

6 Piedmont RL. Spiritual transcendence as a predictor of psychosocial outcome from an outpatient substance abuse program. *Psychol Addict Behav*. 2004; **18**(3): 213–22.

7 Keller RR. Religious diversity in North America. In: Richards PS, Bergin AE, editors. *Handbook of Psychotherapy and Religious Diversity*. Washington, DC: American Psychological Association; 2000. p. 27–55.

8 D'Souza R. Do patients expect psychiatrists to be interested in spiritual issues? *Australas Psychiatry*. 2002; **10**(1): 44–7.

9 Russinova Z, Wewiorski NJ, Cash D. Use of alternative health care practices by persons with serious mental illness: Perceived benefits. *Am J Public Health*. 2002; **92**(10): 1600–3.

10 Flynn PM, Joe GW, Broome KM *et al*. Recovery from opioid addiction in DATOS. *J Subst Abuse Treat*. 2003; **25**(3): 177–86.

11 Lindgren KN, Coursey RD. Spirituality and serious mental illness: a two-part study. *Psychosoc Rehabil J*. 1995; **18**(3): 93–111.

12 Richards PS, Bergin AE. Religious diversity and psychotherapy: conclusions, recommendations, and future directions. In: Richards PS, Bergin AE, editors. *Handbook of Psychotherapy and Religious Diversity*. Washington, DC: American Psychological Association; 2000. p. 469–89.

13 Sue S. In search of cultural competence in psychotherapy and counseling. *Am Psychol*. 1998; **53**(4): 440–8.

14 American Psychiatric Association. *Diagnostic and Statistical Manual of Mental Disorders*. 4th ed, text revision. Washington, DC: American Psychiatric Association; 2000.

15 McCullough JP. *Treatment for Chronic Depression: cognitive behavioral analysis system of psychotherapy*. New York: Guilford Press; 2000.

16 Steketee GS. *Treatment of Obsessive Compulsive Disorder*. New York: Guilford Press; 1996.

17 Klerman GL, Weissman MM, Rounsaville BJ *et al*. *Interpersonal Psychotherapy of Depression*. New York: Basic Books; 1984.

18 Hall GCN. Psychotherapy research with ethnic minorities: empirical, ethical, and conceptual issues. *J Consult Clin Psychol*. 2001; **69**(5): 502–10.

19 Koenig HG. *Handbook of Religion and Mental Health*. San Diego, CA: Academic Press; 1998.

20 Richards PS, Bergin AE. *Handbook of Psychotherapy and Religious Diversity*. Washington, DC: American Psychological Association; 2000.

21 Puchalski CM, Romer AL. Taking a spiritual history allows clinicians to understand patients more fully. *J Palliat Med*. 2000; **3**(1): 129–37.

22 Koenig HP, Pritchett J. Religion and psychotherapy. In: Koenig HG, editor. *Handbook of Religion and Mental Health*. San Diego, CA: Academic Press; 1998. p. 323–36.

23 Koenig HP, Weaver AJ. *Counseling Troubled Older Adults: a handbook for pastors and religious caregivers*. Decatur, GA: Abingdon Press; 1997.

24 Baez A, Hernandez D. Complementary spiritual beliefs in the Latino community: the interface with psychotherapy. *Am J Orthopsychiatry*. 2001; **71**(4): 408–15.

25 Hill PC, Hood RW Jr. *Measures of Religiosity*. Birmingham, AL: Religious Education Press; 1999.

26 Slater W, Hall TW, Edwards KJ. Measuring religion and spirituality: where are we and where are we going? *J Psychol Theol*. 2001; **29**(1): 4–21.

27 Piedmont RL. Does spirituality represent the sixth factor of personality? Spiritual transcendence and the five-factor model. *J Pers.* 1999; **67**(6): 985–1013.

28 Nathan PE, Gorman JM. Efficacy, effectiveness, and the clinical utility of psychotherapy research. In: Nathan PE, Gorman JM, editors. *A Guide to Treatments that Work.* 2nd ed. New York: Oxford University Press; 2002. p. 643–54.

29 MacDonald DA, Holland D. Spirituality and the MMPI-2. *J Clin Psychol.* 2003; **59**(4): 399–410.

30 Sahlein J. When religion enters the dialogue: a guide for practitioners. *Clin Soc Work J.* 2002; **30**(4): 381–401.

31 Greenberg D, Witztum E. The treatment of obsessive-compulsive disorder in strictly religious patients. In: Pato MT, Zohar J, editors. *Current Treatments of Obsessive-Compulsive Disorder.* Washington, DC: American Psychiatric Press; 1991. p. 157–72.

32 Mercer JA. The protestant child, adolescent, and family. *Child Adolesc Psychiatr Clin North Am.* 2004; **13**(1): 161–81.

33 Wilson WP. Religion and psychoses. In: Koenig HG, editor. *Handbook of Religion and Mental Health.* San Diego, CA: Academic Press; 1998. p. 161–73.

34 Tek C, Ulug B. Religiosity and religious obsessions in obsessive-compulsive disorder. *Psychiatry Res.* 2001; **104**(2): 99–108.

35 Jerrell JM, Shugart MA. A comparison of the phenomenology and treatment of youths and adults with bipolar I disorder in a state mental health system. *J Affect Disord.* 2004; **80**(1): 29–35.

36 Murphy PE, Ciarrocchi JW, Piedmont RL *et al.* The relation of religious belief and practices, depression, and hopelessness in persons with clinical depression. *J Consult Clin Psychol.* 2000; **68**(6): 1102–6.

37 Baetz M, Larson DB, Marcoux G *et al.* Canadian psychiatric inpatient religious commitment: an association with mental health. *Can J Psychiatry.* 2002; **47**(2): 159–66.

38 Herrenkohl TI, Tajima EA, Whitney SD *et al.* Protection against antisocial behavior in children exposed to physically abusive discipline. *J Adolesc Health.* 2005; **36**(6): 457–65.

39 Koenig HG. Religion, spirituality, and medicine: research findings and implications for clinical practice. *South Med J.* 2004; **97**(12): 1194–200.

40 Tepper L, Rogers SA, Coleman EM *et al.* The prevalence of religious coping among persons with persistent mental illness. *Psychiatr Serv.* 2001; **52**(5): 660–5.

41 Levin JS, Larson DB, Puchalski CM. Religion and spirituality in medicine: research and education. *JAMA.* 1997; **278**(9): 792–3.

42 Levin JS, Chatters LM. Research on religion and mental health: an overview of empirical findings and theoretical issues. In: Koenig HG, editor. *Handbook of Religion and Mental Health.* San Diego, CA: Academic Press; 1998. p. 33–50.

43 Gartner J, Larson DB, Allen GD. Religious commitment and mental health: a review of the empirical literature. *J Psychol Theol.* 1991; **19**(1): 6–25.

44 Azhar MZ, Varma SL, Dharap AS. Religious psychotherapy in anxiety disorder patients. *Acta Psychiatr Scand.* 1994; **90**(1): 1–3.

45 Chambless DL, Ollendick TH. Empirically supported psychological interventions: controversies and evidence. *Annu Rev Psychol.* 2001; **52**: 685–716.

46 Propst LR, Ostrom R, Watkins P et al. Comparative efficacy of religious and nonreligious cognitive-behavioral therapy for the treatment of clinical depression in religious individuals. *J Consult Clin Psychol.* 1992; **60**(1): 94–103.

47 Miller WR, Rollnick S. *Motivational Interviewing: preparing people for change.* New York: Guilford Press; 2002.

48 Beck AT, Rush AJ, Shaw BF et al. *Cognitive Therapy of Depression: a treatment manual.* New York: Guilford Press; 1979.

Notes to Chapter 6: Children and Families from Diverse Backgrounds

1 Brestan EV, Eyberg SM. Effective psychosocial treatments of conduct disordered children and adolescents: 29 years, 82 studies, and 5,272 kids. *J Clin Child Psychol.* 1998; **27**(2): 180–9.

2 Kumpfer KL, Alvarado R. *Effective Family Strengthening Interventions.* Washington, DC: Office of Juvenile Justice and Delinquency Prevention; 1998.

3 Sanders MR. New directions in behavioral family intervention with children: from clinical management to prevention. *N Z J Psychol.* 1992; **21**(1): 25–36.

4 Webster-Stratton C, Hammond M. Predictors of treatment outcome in parent training for families with conduct problem children. *Behav Ther.* 1990; **21**(3): 319–37.

5 Barkley RA. *Defiant Children: a clinician's manual for assessment and parent training.* 2nd ed. New York: Guilford Press; 1997.

6 Forehand R, Long N. *Parenting the Strong-Willed Child: the clinically proven five-week program for parents of two- to six-year-olds.* Chicago: Contemporary Books; 1996.

7 Sue S. In search of cultural competence in psychotherapy and counseling. *Am Psychol.* 1998; **53**(4): 440–8.

8 Conners CK. *Conners' Rating Scales-Revised Technical Manual.* North Tonawanda, NY: Multi-Health Systems; 1997.

9 Dupaul GJ, Power TJ, Anastopoulos AD et al. *ADHD Rating Scale-IV: checklist, norms, and clinical interpretation.* New York: Guilford Press; 1998.

10 Achenbach TM. *Manual for the Child Behavior Checklist/4–18 and 1991 Profile.* Burlington, VT: University of Vermont, Department of Psychiatry; 1991.

11 Forehand R, Kotchick BA. Cultural diversity: a wake-up call for parent training. *Behav Ther.* 1996; **27**(2): 187–206.

12 Lambert MC, Rowan GT, Lyubansky M et al. Do problems of clinic-referred African-American children overlap with the CBCL? *J Child Fam Stud.* 2002; **11**(3): 271–85.

13 Weisz JR, Weiss B, Somsong S *et al*. Syndromal structure of psychopathology in children of Thailand and the United States. *J Consult Clin Psychol*. 2003; **71**(2): 375–85.

14 McDermott D. Parenting and ethnicity. In: Fine MJ, Lee SW, editors. *Handbook of Diversity in Parent Education: the changing faces of parenting and parent education*. San Diego, CA: Academic Press; 2001. p. 73–96.

15 Pinderhughes EE, Dodge KA, Bates JE *et al*. Discipline responses: influences of parents' socioeconomic status, ethnicity, beliefs about parenting, stress, and cognitive-emotional processes. *J Fam Psychol*. 2000; **14**(3): 380–400.

16 Eamon MK. Poverty, parenting, peer, and neighborhood influences on young adolescent antisocial behavior. *J Soc Serv Res*. 2001; **28**(1): 1–23.

17 Ogbu JU. A cultural ecology of competence among inner-city blacks. In: Spencer MB, Brookins GK, Allen WR, editors. *Beginnings: the social and affective development of black children*. Hillsdale, NJ: Lawrence Erlbaum; 1985. p. 45–66.

18 Yao EL. Adjustment needs of Asian immigrant children. *Elementary Sch Guid Couns*. 1985; **19**(3): 222–7.

19 Middlemiss W. Brief report: poverty, stress, and support: patterns of parenting behaviour among lower income black and lower income white mothers. *Infant Child Dev*. 2003; **12**(3): 293–300.

20 Strain PS, Young CC, Horowitz J. Generalized behavior change during oppositional child training: an examination of child and family demographic variables. *Behav Modif*. 1981; **5**(1): 15–26.

21 Sue DW, Sue D. *Counseling the Culturally Different: theory and practice*. 2nd ed. Oxford: John Wiley & Sons; 1990.

22 Straus MA, Stewart JH. Corporal punishment by American parents: national data on prevalence, chronicity, severity, and duration, in relation to child and family characteristics. *Clin Child Fam Psychol Rev*. 1999; **2**(2): 55–70.

23 Lindahl KM. Family process variables and children's disruptive behavior problems. *J Fam Psychol*. 1998; **12**(3): 420–36.

24 Patterson GR, Dishion TJ. Contributions of families and peers to delinquency. *Criminology*. 1985; **23**(1): 63–79.

25 Forehand R, Kotchick BA. Behavioral parent training: current challenges and potential solutions. *J Child Fam Stud*. 2002; **11**(4): 377–84.

26 Capage LC, Bennett GM, McNeil CB. A comparison between African American and Caucasian children referred for treatment of disruptive behavior disorders. *Child Fam Behav Ther*. 2001; **23**(1): 1–14.

27 Reid MJ, Webster-Stratton C, Beauchaine TP. Parent training in Head Start: a comparison of program response among African American, Asian American, Caucasian, and Hispanic mothers. *Prev Sci*. 2001; **2**(4): 209–27.

28 Bradley RH, Corwyn RF, McAdoo HP *et al*. The home environments of children in the United States. Part I: variations by age, ethnicity, and poverty status. *Child Dev*. 2001; **72**(6): 844–67.

29 McMahon RJ, Forehand R, Griest DL *et al*. Who drops out of treatment during parent behavioral training? *Behav Couns Q*. 1981; **1**(1): 79–85.

30 Dumas JE. Child, adult-interactional, and socioeconomic setting events as predictors of parent training outcome. *Educ Treat Child.* 1984; **7**(4): 351–64.

31 MacKenzie EP, Fite PJ, Bates JE. Predicting outcome in behavioral parent training: expected and unexpected results. *Child Fam Behav Ther.* 2004; **26**(2): 37–53.

32 Kotchick BA, Forehand R. Putting parenting practices in perspective: a discussion of the contextual factors that shape parenting practice. *J Child Fam Stud.* 2002; **11**(3): 255–69.

33 Heffer RW, Kelley ML. Mothers' acceptance of behavioral interventions for children: the influence of parent race and income. *Behav Ther.* 1987; **2**: 153–63.

34 Eamon MK, Venkataraman M. Implementing parent management training in the context of poverty. *Am J Fam Ther.* 2003; **31**(4): 281–93.

35 Karpowitz DH. American families in the 1990s and beyond. In: Fine MJ, Lee SW, editors. *Handbook of Diversity in Parent Education: the changing faces of parenting and parent education.* San Diego, CA: Academic Press; 2001. p. 1–14.

36 Meyers SA. Adapting parent education programs to meet the needs of fathers: an ecological perspective. *Fam Relat.* 1993; **42**: 447–52.

37 Sirridge ST. Parent education for fathers. In: Fine MJ, Lee SW, editors. *Handbook of Diversity in Parent Education: the changing faces of parenting and parent education.* San Diego, CA: Academic Press; 2001. p. 179–97.

38 Adesso VJ, Lipson JW. Group training of parents as therapists for their children. *Behav Ther.* 1981; **12**(5): 625–33.

39 Webster-Stratton C, Kolpacoff M, Hollinsworth T. Self-administered videotape therapy for families with conduct-problem children: comparison with two cost-effective treatments and a control group. *J Consult Clin Psychol.* 1988; **56**(4): 558–66.

40 McBride BA. Parent education and support programs for fathers: outcome effects on paternal involvement. *Early Child Dev Care.* 1991; **67**: 73–85.

41 Young MH, Dawson TJ. Perception of child difficulty and levels of depression in caregiving grandmothers. *J Ment Health Aging.* 2003; **9**(2): 111–22.

42 Landry-Meyer L. Research into action: recommended intervention strategies for grandparent caregivers. *Fam Relat.* 1999; **48**(4): 381–9.

43 Burton LM. Black grandparents rearing children of drug-addicted parents: stressors, outcomes, and social service needs. *Gerontologist.* 1992; **32**(6): 744–51.

44 Fuller-Thomson E, Minkler M. The mental and physical health of grandmothers who are raising their grandchildren. *J Ment Health Aging.* 2000; **6**(4): 311–23.

45 Burnette D. Physical and emotional well-being of custodial grandparents in Latino families. *Am J Orthopsychiatry.* 1999; **69**(3): 305–18.

46 Henggeler SW, Schoenwald SK, Borduin CM *et al. Multisystemic Treatment of Antisocial Behavior in Children and Adolescents.* New York: Guilford Press; 1998.

47 Alexander JF, Parsons BV. *Functional Family Therapy.* Monterey, CA: Brooks/Cole; 1982.

48 Henggeler SW, Sheidow AJ. Conduct disorder and delinquency. *J Marital Fam Ther.* 2003; **29**(4): 505–22.

49 Sheidow AJ, Henggeler SW, Schoenwald SK. Multisystemic therapy. In: Sexton TL, Weeks GR et al, editors. *Handbook of Family Therapy: the science and practice of working with families and couples*. New York: Brunner-Routledge; 2003. p. 303–22.

50 American Psychological Association. Guidelines on multicultural education, training, research, practice, and organizational change for psychologists. *Am Psychol*. 2003; **58**(5): 377–402.

Notes to Chapter 7: Individuals with Dual Diagnosis

1 Reiss S, Levitan GW, Szyszko J. Diagnostic overshadowing and professional experience with retarded persons. *Am J Ment Defic*. 1982; **87**: 396–402.

2 Reiss S. People with a dual diagnosis: America's powerless population. In: Tymchuk AJ, Lakin CJ, Luckasson R, editors. *The Forgotten Generation: the status and challenges of adults with mild cognitive limitations*. Baltimore, MD: Paul H. Brooks Publishing Co; 2001. p. 275–98.

3 American Psychiatric Association. *Diagnostic and Statistical Manual of Mental Disorders*. 4th ed. Washington DC: American Psychiatric Association; 1994.

4 American Psychiatric Association. *Diagnostic and Statistical Manual of Mental Disorders*. 4th ed, text revision. Washington DC: American Psychiatric Association; 2000.

5 Cullinan D, Epstein M, Olinger, E. School behavior problems of mentally retarded and normal females. *Ment Retard Learn Disabil Bull*. 1983; **11**: 104–9.

6 Nezu CM, Nezu AM, Gill-Weiss MJ. *Psychopathology in Persons with Mental Retardation: clinical guidelines for assessment and treatment*. Champaign, IL: Research Press; 1992.

7 Goldberg B, Gitta MZ, Puddephatt A. Personality and trait disturbances in an adult mental retardation population: significance for psychiatric management. *J Intellect Disabil Res*. 1995; **39**: 284–94.

8 Bradley EA, Summers JA, Wood HL *et al*. Comparing rates of psychiatric and behavior disorders in adolescents and young adults with severe intellectual disability with and without autism. *J Autism Dev Disord*. 2004; **34**: 151–61.

9 Ghaziuddin M, Weidmer-Mikhail E, Ghaziuddin N. Comorbidity of Asperger syndrome: a preliminary report. *J Intellect Disabil Res*. 1998; **42**: 279–83.

10 Rutter M, Tizard J, Yule W *et al*. Isle of Wight studies, 1964–1974. *Psychol Med*. 1976; **6**: 313–32.

11 Kessler RC, Chiu WT, Demler O *et al*. Prevalence, severity, and comorbidity of twelve-month DSM-IV disorders in the National Comorbidity Survey Replication (NCS-R). *Arch Gen Psychiatry*. 2005; **62**: 617–27.

12 Ghaziuddin M. Asperger syndrome: Associated psychiatric and medical conditions. *Focus Autism Dev Disabil*. 2002; **17**: 138–44.

13 Borthwick-Duffy SA. Epidemiology and prevalence of psychopathology in people with mental retardation. *J Consult Clin Psychol*. 1994; **62**: 17–27.

14 Jacobson JW. Problem behavior and psychiatric impairment within a developmentally disabled population: III psychotropic medication. *Res Dev Disabil*. 1988; **9**: 23–38.

15 Reiss S. Prevalence of dual diagnosis in community-based day programs in the Chicago metropolitan area. *Am J Ment Retard*. 1990; **94**: 578–85.

16 Reiss S, Levitan GW, McNally RJ. Emotionally disturbed mentally retarded people: an underserved population. *Am Psychol*. 1982; **37**: 361–7.

17 Moss SC. Methodological issues in the diagnosis of psychiatric disorders in adults with learning disabilities. *Thornfield J (University of Dublin)*. 1995; **18**: 9–18.

18 Nisbett R, Ross L. *Human Inference: strategies and shortcomings of social judgment*. Englewood Cliffs, NJ: Prentice-Hall; 1980.

19 Nelson-Gray RO. Treatment utility of psychological assessment. *Psychol Assess*. 2003; **15**: 521–31.

20 Szymanski LS, King B, Goldberg B *et al*. Diagnosis of mental disorders in people with mental retardation. In: Reiss S, Aman MG, editors. *Psychotropic Medication and Developmental Disabilities: the international consensus handbook*. Columbus, OH: The Ohio State University (Distributed by the American Association on Mental Retardation); 1998.

21 Sue S. In search of cultural competence in psychotherapy and counseling. *Am Psychol*. 1998; **53**: 440–8.

22 Kazdin AE. Developmental psychopathology. Current research, issues, and directions. *Am Psychol*. 1989; **44**: 180–7.

23 Garber J. Classification of childhood psychopathology: a developmental perspective. *Child Dev*. 1984; **55**: 30–48.

24 McCullough JP Jr. *Treatment for Chronic Depression: cognitive behavioral analysis system of psychotherapy (CBASP)*. New York: Guilford Press; 2000.

25 Sevin JA, Bowers-Stephens C, Hamilton ML *et al*. Integrating behavioral and pharmacological interventions in treating clients with psychiatric disorders and mental retardation. *Res Dev Disabil*. 2001; **22**: 463–85.

26 Reid WH. *The Treatment of Psychiatric Disorders*. New York: Brunner/Mazel; 1989.

27 Aman MG. *Assessing Psychopathology and Behaviour Problems in Persons with Mental Retardation*. Rockville, MD: US Department of Health and Human Services; 1991.

28 Reiss S. Assessment of psychopathology in persons with mental retardation. In: Maison JL, Barrett RP, editors. *Psychopathology in the Mentally Retarded*. 2nd ed. Needham Heights, MA: Allyn & Bacon; 1993. p. 17–40.

29 Rush KS, Bowman LG, Eidman SL *et al*. Assessing psychopathology in individuals with developmental disabilities. *Behav Modif*. 2004; **28**: 621–37.

30 Matson JL. *The PIMRA Manual*. Orlando Park, IL: International Diagnostic Systems; 1988.

31 Matson JL, Coe DA, Gardner WI *et al*. A factor analytic study of the diagnostic assessment for the severely handicapped scale. *J Nerv Ment Dis*. 1991; **179**: 553–7.

32 Reiss S. The Reiss screen for maladaptive behavior test manual. Worthington, OH: IDS Publishing Corporation; 1988.

33 Moss SC, Prosser H, Costello H *et al*. Reliability and validity of the PAS-ADD checklist for detecting psychiatric disorders in adults with intellectual disabilities. *J Intellect Disabil Res*. 1998; **42**: 173–83.

34 Aman MG, Singh NM. Psychometric characteristics of the aberrant behavior checklist. *Am J Ment Defic*. 1985; **89**: 492–502.

35 Sturmy P, Reed J, Corbett J. Psychometric assessment of psychiatric disorders in people with learning disabilities (mental handicap): a review of measures. *Psychol Med*. 1991; **21**: 143–55.

36 Sabatino DA, Vance HB, Miller TL. Defining best diagnostic practices. In: Vance HB, editor. *Best Practices in Assessment for School and Clinical Settings*. Brandon, VT: Clinical Psychology Press; 1993. p. 1–28.

37 Green CW, Reid DH. Defining, validating, and increasing indices of happiness among people with profound multiple disabilities. *J Appl Behav Anal*. 1996; **29**: 67–78.

38 Green CW, Gardner SM, Reid DH. Increasing indices of happiness among people with profound multiple disabilities: a program replication and component analysis. *J Appl Behav Anal*. 1997; **30**: 217–28.

39 Green CW, Reid DH. Reducing indices of unhappiness among individuals with profound multiple disabilities during therapeutic exercise routines. *J Appl Behav Anal*. 1999; **32**: 137–48.

40 Rush KS, Crockett JL, Hagopian LP. An analysis of the selective effects of NCR with punishment targeting screaming and SIB associated with positive affect. *Behav Interv*. 2001; **16**: 127–35.

41 Toole LM, Bowman LG, Thomason J *et al*. Observed increases in positive affect during a levels treatment. *Behav Interv*. 2003; **18**: 35–42.

42 Masi G, Favilla L, Mucci M. Generalized anxiety disorder in adolescents and young adults with mental retardation. *Psychiatry Interpers Biol Process*. 2000; **63**: 54–64.

43 Deb S, Thomas M, Bright C. Mental disorder in adults with intellectual disability 2: the rate of behaviour disorders among a community-based population aged between 16 and 64 years. *J Intellect Disabil Res*. 2001; **45**: 506–14.

44 Benson BA. Psychological interventions for people with intellectual disability and mental health problems. *Curr Opin Psychiatry*. 2004; **17**: 353–7.

45 Nathan PE, Gorman JM. Efficacy, effectiveness, and the clinical utility of psychotherapy research. In: Nathan PE, Gorman JM, editors. *A Guide to Treatments that Work*. New York: Oxford University Press; 2002. p. 643–54.

46 Prout HT, Nowak-Drabik KM. Psychotherapy with persons who have mental retardation: an evaluation of effectiveness. *Am J Ment Retard*. 2003; **108**: 83–93.

47 Beail N. What works for people with mental retardation? Critical commentary on cognitive-behavioral and psychodynamic psychotherapy research. *Ment Retard*. 2003; **41**: 468–72.

48 Summers SJ. Psychological intervention for people with learning disabilities who have experienced bereavement: a case study illustration. *Br J Learn Disabil.* 2003; **31**: 46–53.

49 Newman C, Adams K. Dog gone good: managing dog phobia in a teenage boy with a learning disability. *Br J Learn Disabil.* 2004; **31**: 46–53.

50 Van Orden K, Wingate LR, Gordon KH *et al.* Interpersonal factors as vulnerability for psychopathology over the life course. In: Hankin BL, Abela J, editors. *Development of Psychopathology: a vulnerability-stress perspective.* San Diego, CA: Sage Publications; 2005. p. 136–60.

51 Butzer B, Konstantareas MM. Depression, temperament, and their relationship to other characteristics in children with Asperger's disorder. *J Dev Disabil.* 2003; **10**: 67–72.

52 Smith C. Using social stories to enhance behaviour in children with autistic spectrum difficulties. *Educ Psychol Prac.* 2001; **17**: 337–45.

53 Lovaas OI. Behavioral treatment and normal educational and intellectual functioning in young autistic children. *J Consult Clin Psychol.* 1987; **55**: 3–9.

54 McEachin JJ, Smith T, Lovaas OI. Long-term outcome for children who received early intensive behavioral treatment. *Am J Ment Retard.* 1993; **97**: 359–72.

55 Cardaciotto L, Herbert JD. Cognitive behavior therapy for social anxiety disorder in the context of Asperger's syndrome: a single-subject report. *Cogn Behav Prac.* 2004; **11**: 75–81.

Notes to Chapter 8: *Summary and Future Directions*

1 Sue S. In search of cultural competence in psychotherapy and counseling. *Am Psychol.* 1998; **53**(4): 440–8.

2 Puchalski CM, Romer AL. Taking a spiritual history allows clinicians to understand patients more fully. *J Palliat Med.* 2000; **3**: 129–37.

3 Koenig HG, Pritchett J. Religion and psychotherapy. In: Koenig H, editor. *Handbook of Religion and Mental Health.* San Diego, CA: Academic Press; 1998. p. 323–36.

4 Anandarajah G, Hight E. Spirituality and medical practice: using HOPE questions as a practical tool for spiritual assessment. *Am Fam Physician.* 2001; **63**: 81–8.

5 Richards PS, Bergin AE. *Handbook of Psychotherapy and Religious Diversity.* Washington, DC: American Psychological Association; 2000.

6 Alvidrez J, Azocar F, Miranda J. Demystifying the concept of ethnicity for psychotherapy researchers. *J Consult Clin Psychol.* 1996; **64**: 903–8.

7 Altarriba J, Santiago-Rivera AL. Current perspectives on using linguistic and cultural factors in counseling the Hispanic client. *Prof Psychol Res Pract.* 1994; **25**: 388–97.

8 American Psychological Association. Guidelines for providers of psychological services to ethnic, linguistic, and culturally diverse populations. *Am Psychol.* 1993; **48**: 458.

9   Hall GC. Psychotherapy research with ethnic minorities: empirical, ethical, and conceptual issues. *J Consult Clin Psychol.* 2001; **69**: 502–10.

10 O'Reardon JP, Ringel DL, Dinges DF *et al.* Circadian eating and sleeping pattern in the night eating syndrome. *Obes Res.* 2004; **12**: 1789–96.

11 Streigel-Moore RH, Dohm F, Hook JM *et al.* Night eating syndrome in young adult women: prevalence and correlates. *Int J Eat Disord.* 2005; **37**: 200–6.

12 Avalon L, Young MA. A comparison of depressive symptoms in African Americans and Caucasian Americans. *J Cross Cult Psychol.* 2003; **34**(1): 111–24.

13 Westen D, Harnden-Fischer J. Personality profiles in eating disorders: rethinking the distinction between Axis I and Axis II. *Am J Psychiatry.* 2001; **158**: 547–62.

14 Chambless DL, Hollon SD. Defining empirically supported therapies. *J Consult Clin Psychol.* 1998; **66**: 7–18.

15 Malgady RG, Rogler LH, Costantino G. Hero/heroine modeling for Puerto Rican adolescents: a preventive mental health intervention. *J Consult Clin Psychol.* 1990; **58**: 469–74.

16 Wells K, Sherbourne C, Schoenbaum M *et al.* Five-year impact of quality improvement for depression: results of a group-level randomized controlled trial. *Arch Gen Psychiatry.* 2004; **61**: 378–86.

17 Pina AA, Silverman WK, Fuentes RM *et al.* Exposure-based cognitive-behavioral treatment for phobic and anxiety disorders: treatment effects and maintenance for Hispanic/Latino relative to European-American youths. *J Am Acad Child Adolesc Psychiatry.* 2003; **42**: 1179–87.

18 Treadwell KRH, Flannery-Schroeder EC, Kendall PC. Ethnicity and gender in relation to adaptive functioning, diagnostic status, and treatment outcome in children from an anxiety clinic. *J Anxiety Disord.* 1995; **9**: 373–84.

19 Brown C, Schulberg HC, Sacco D *et al.* Effectiveness of treatments for major depression in primary medical care practice: a post hoc analysis of outcomes for African American and White patients. *J Affect Disord.* 1999; **53**: 185–92.

20 Beck AT, Rush AJ, Shaw BF *et al. Cognitive Therapy of Depression.* New York: Guilford Press; 1979.

21 Klerman GL, Weissman MM, Rounsaville BJ *et al. Interpersonal Psychotherapy of Depression.* New York: Basic Books; 1984.

22 McCullough JP Jr. *Treatment for Chronic Depression: cognitive behavioral analysis system of psychotherapy.* New York: Guilford Press; 2000.

23 Garnet L, Hancock KA, Cochran SD *et al.* Issues in psychotherapy with lesbians and gay men: a survey of psychologists. *Am Psychol.* 1991; **46**: 964–72.

24 Russinova Z, Wewiorski NJ, Cash D. Use of alternative health care practices by persons with serious mental illness: perceived benefits. *Am J Public Health.* 2002; **92**: 1600–3.

25 United States Department of Health and Human Services. *Mental Health: culture, race, and ethnicity – a supplement to mental health: a report of the surgeon general – executive summary.* Rockville, MD: US Department of Health and Human Services, Public Health Service, Office of the Surgeon General, 2001.

26 Gallo JJ, Marino S, Ford D *et al*. Filters on the pathway to mental health care: sociodemographic factors. *Psychol Med*. 1995; **25**: 1149–60.
27 Vega WA, Warheit G, Buhl-Auth J *et al*. The prevalence of depressive symptoms among Mexican Americans and Anglos. *Am J Epidemiol*. 1984; **120**: 592–607.
28 Vega WA, Kolody B, Aguilar-Gaxiola S *et al*. Gaps in services utilization by Mexican Americans with mental health problems. *Am J Psychiatry*. 1999; **156**: 928–34.
29 Miranda J, Cooper LA. Disparities in care for depression among primary care patients. *J Gen Intern Med*. 2004; **19**: 120–6.

Index

grandparents 81, 83, 85–6, 88–9, 92–3, 95, 97
Green, CW 110, 120
Greenberg, D 72
grief 66, 113
group therapy 18, 19
guardians 81, 88, 94
guilt 72, 75, 78

Hall, GCN 4, 20
hallucinations 66
Hammond, M 90
hand-washing rituals 72, 76, 78
happiness 110, 120
hate crimes 48
health insurance 3–4, 10, 30, 126
Hegna, K 52
herbal remedies 32, 86
Hernandez, D 70
Hight, E 70
Hill, PC 63, 71
Hispanic Stress Inventory 14
Hispanic/Latino clients 9–24
    case illustration 20–3
    clinical observations 11–14
        assessment 11
        diagnosis 12
        treatment 12–14
    diverse families 88, 92, 93, 95
    future directions 24
    mental health services 1, 3–4, 7, 122, 125,
    126
    overview 9–11
    research literature 14–20
        assessment 14–16
        diagnosis 16–17
        treatment 18–20
home token economy 82, 87, 89
homophobia 44, 52, 53
homosexuality 43–6, 47–50, 61, 124 see also
    lesbian, gay and bisexual clients
Hood, RW Jr 71
Hooker, E 44
HOPE (hope, organized religion, personal
    practices, effects) 70, 71
hopelessness 72
hospitalization 66, 72
human judgment see judgment of clinician
hyperactivity 86 see also attention-deficit
    hyperactivity disorder
hyper-religiosity 72
hypertension 73
hypomania 34
hypotheses
    African American clients 29
    cultural competence 6, 8
    dual diagnosis 106

Hispanic/Latino clients 11
LGB clients 48
mental health services 121, 122, 123, 124

identity 19, 47, 53, 60
immigration history 14, 24, 122
impulse control disorders 102
income 2, 3, 17, 29–30, 34
infidelity 21–2, 75–9
informed consent 26, 112
inpatient services 25, 26, 66
insomnia 107
insurance 3–4, 10, 30, 126
intellectual disabilities 111, 112, 113
intelligence tests 26, 27, 34–5
Interpersonal Psychotherapy (IPT)
    African American clients 37
    Hispanic/Latino clients 18, 24
    LGB clients 50
    mental health services treatment 125
    religiously diverse clients 68, 76, 78
interpersonal relationships
    dual diagnosis 113, 114, 118
    Hispanic/Latino clients 10, 13, 14, 23, 24
    mental health services treatment 125
interpreters 15, 122
interviews
    diverse families 86, 89
    dual diagnosis 104, 105, 106, 114
    Hispanic/Latino clients 15
    religiously diverse clients 65
IPT see Interpersonal Psychotherapy
IQ (intelligence quotient) tests 27, 34–5

Jerrell, JM 72
Judaism 65
judgment of clinician
    dual diagnosis 104
    LGB clients 57
    religiously diverse clients 67–9, 76, 79
    scientific mindedness 6, 123

Kinsey, Alfred 48
knowledge 5–6
Koenig, HG 69
Koening, HP 70
Kotchick, BA 91

language
    African American clients 36
    cultural competence 4, 5
    dual diagnosis 103–4
    Hispanic/Latino clients 10–11, 14–16,
        19–20, 22, 24, 122
Latino clients 3, 9, 17, 87 see also Hispanic/
    Latino clients